Rx FOR HOSPITALS

Rx FOR HOSPITALS

NEW HOPE FOR MEDICARE IN THE NINETIES

PHILIP HASSEN
WITH SHARON LINDENBURGER

Stoddart

First published in 1993 by
Stoddart Publishing Co. Limited
34 Lesmill Road
Toronto, Canada
M3B 2T6
(416) 445-3333

Canadian Cataloguing in Publication Data

Hassen, Philip
    Rx for hospitals: new hope for medicare in the nineties

Includes index.
ISBN 0-7737-2700-0

1. Hospitals - Canada - Business management.
2. Hospitals - Canada - Finance. 3. Insurance, Health -
Canada. I. Title.

RA971.3.H3 1993   338.4'336211'0971   C93-09313

Printed and bound in Canada

*Stoddart Publishing gratefully acknowledges the support
of the Canada Council, Ontario Ministry of Culture,
Tourism, and Recreation, Ontario Arts Council, and
Ontario Publishing Centre in the development of writing
and publishing in Canada.*

Contents

Foreword

I must go on a diet . . . tomorrow."

We have the best of intentions. Who doesn't? And who is unfamiliar with the earnest laying of plans to carry out those intentions? My bookshelf is full of pamphlets and guidebooks on weight loss and exercise. Ten New Year's Eves have come and gone, each with serious resolutions to get started toward fitness. Many times have I begun the regimen — four days in a row of four-mile jogs, a pantry shelf stocked with help: "A complete meal in a can — substitute one for breakfast and one for lunch, and watch those extra inches melt off!"

But the bathroom scale tells the truth. It reads no books, jogs no jogs, and drinks nothing as a substitute; it just tells me what I have done. "You have made no changes," it says.

"What do you mean?" I rebut. "Look at all those changes! Last Tuesday I ran, drank a meal in a can, and tomorrow I may do it all over again. You're wrong, scale; you *must* be wrong."

"No changes," the scale says. "No changes at all."

When we love something, we change. My wife and I love hiking in the wilderness, and no month passes without a pilgrimage to our favourite local outdoor equipment store. We are there in search of change. A backpack with a novel design catches our eye; we try it on. If we like it, we buy it; and then we use it. A hundred days we have hiked in the North Cascades of Washington — our favourite terrain — and yet we are among the first to buy a new book on that region; it hints of a new trail yet untried, or a few interesting details on an old one.

Through change we intend improvement. In my years of acquaintance with "quality management," only recently has it come clear to me how intimate is the relationship between change and improvement. Indeed, I now believe that, for practical purposes, *little useful improvement occurs without the self-conscious introduction of change.* But the self-conscious introduction of change is extremely difficult. That is how love and change come to be related: sometimes it takes the energy of love to generate the courage to change. (The energy of fear can also work; but the energy of love is better.)

Of course, change occurs often without improvement. In fact, change is constant. We react, struggling for stability. How much of the energy of leaders in the modern health care system is absorbed in that struggle! They seem so often now like that heroic captain, fists tightly wrapped on the wheel in gale-force winds, cheeks red and wet with waves breaking over the helm, leaning with all his might to hold the ship on course. The change is from without, and the struggle is to remain the same.

That is not love of the sort that sends me hiking on mountains. It is not striving for a new future; it is holding on.

The key difference is this: one way seeks stability, the other seeks growth. One way resists changes from outside; the other introduces changes from within. One way finds the past good enough; the other aims in a new direction. One captain holds the course; the other changes course.

Holding the course is not what health care needs in the United States or in Canada. It is not good enough. In our well-intended hands, people die who could have been saved. Our current best efforts at work contain levels of waste, inefficiency, and complexity that drain resources from other social investments. Our patients and their families reasonably rely on us for consistency, dignity, safety, answers to their questions, and reduction of their pain, and far too often we let them down. In the United States, especially, inequities in health status among races and socio-economic groups persist and offend conscience. If we accept in the future what we have been in the past, it would be hard to be proud.

Total quality management enters health care as an approach worth learning, and this book explores the ideas and experiences of some of its most able practitioners in all of health care. The reader can learn a lot about TQM from careful study of this book.

Although Dr. W. Edwards Deming rejects labelling his work, many of us use the expression to refer, at least in part, to Deming's framework of elements of knowledge that can better equip subject-matter experts — such as surgeons, nurses, or administrators — to improve their work and its effects. The categories of knowledge, which together we might call TQM, are these:

(a) *Knowledge of the System.* Since most important qualities or results derive from complex interactions among elements of a system with a common aim, it is important to understand the key properties of such complex systems. Questions arise like these: What are our common aims? (Hence TQM's focus on mission, vision, values, and constancy.) To whom or what am I connected? Of what am I a part? (Hence TQM's use of tools, like flow charts, that allow people to visualize the system as a whole.) What are the dynamics of complex systems — which often contain counter-intuitive delays and oscillations, confounding usual views of cause-and-effect?

b) *Knowledge of Variation.* The more we know about how a system functions, the better we will identify plausible improvements. The better we can interpret data on variation, the more sensible we can be in acting in response to such data. The would-be "improver" lives in a world of information; and the ability to collect and digest information is inseparable from the improvement process.

(c) *An Approach to Increasing Knowledge.* Sound, efficient improvement involves learning, especially in a scientific mode in which good ideas are clarified and tested and the results of the tests are correctly interpreted and used. The Plan-Do-Check-Act cycle (the "Shewhart Cycle") is at the very heart of the theory of learning in TQM. We improve by trying sensible changes and learning from the trials, and this involves both attitudes and skills in learning.

(d) *An Approach to Psychology.* People are fundamentally different from all other "resources" in a complex system. (In fact, Peter Senge wonders whether the term "human resources" is basically misleading.) Only people can create and embrace purposes; and it is in the spirit and skill of people that the opportunity for wide-scale improvement lies. Therefore, Deming reminds us, our beliefs about people, even if we never actually state them, matter a great deal in the effectiveness of efforts to improve. Why do people do what they do? How do they learn, and vary in their approach to learning? How do they act in groups, and why? How do conflicts of aim or opinion get identified and resolved?

This framework of elements of knowledge for improvement is as powerful as any I know, and yet we are left with one disabling observation as we watch this framework, in its various vocabularies, enter the health care world: namely, *despite growing knowledge of the framework of TQM methods, health care is not yet changing*. The great challenge before the masters of TQM in health care, masters such as the author of this book, is to see clearly what stands today between the marvelous, moving, fascinating intellectual framework that is TQM in any disciplined form, and the actual day-to-day experiences that, collectively, *are* the health care system.

We do not, after all, seek TQM; we seek changes in the system we love. I do not seek trips to the local outdoor equipment store; I seek better mountain hiking. From the changes I make, you can tell how much I care.

The test of our commitment to improving health care will not be in our willingness to learn a new method; it will be in our willingness to make and test actual changes in our real work, and then to act based on what we have learned. Our success in improvement will lie in the *intersection* of these newfound and powerful methods, on the one hand, and the *actual* work we do on the other. If work does not change — if *we* do not change it — then TQM will be judged a fad, guaranteed. Should that happen, the sad error will not have been in total quality management, but in our commitment to change.

DONALD M. BERWICK, M.D.

Acknowledgements

Foremost may I thank everyone who works at St. Joseph's Health Centre, London, for their trust in me to lead them where few have gone; for their optimism and commitment to our shared vision of a better tomorrow; and for their deep commitment to change so we may improve how we serve each other and most importantly our patients, residents, and the community. Many assisted and encouraged me but none more than Jane Parkinson, our Director of Quality Management, my personal mentor. Some of those who also committed time to the book were Peter Cordy, M.D., Paul Cooper, M.D., Peggy Roffey, Amy Lee, Sarah DeKay, Nancy Cordell, Sheila Davis, and Helen MacKenzie.

The Board of St. Joseph's Health Centre supported and encouraged the writing of this book, and I am also grateful to the Health Centre's vice-presidents who were willing to go the extra mile in ensuring that the Centre's needs were being attended to, making it possible for me to devote time to this recounting of St. Joseph's quality journey.

As well, I would like to thank Donald G. Bastian of Stoddart Publishing for his encouragement, unfailing patience, and good humour in guiding me, Sharon Lindenburger, and the manuscript through the complexities of the publishing process.

Most important of all, I thank my family for enduring with me the ups and downs of this time-consuming, yet enormously exciting journey.

PHILIP HASSEN

Introduction

*R*x *for Hospitals* is meant to inject some hope into the gloomy tone of debate concerning Canada's health care system and, in particular, its hospitals. In the few decades since health care became publicly funded and universally accessible, it has rapidly entrenched itself in the minds and hearts of Canadians as a fundamental value, or even right, of all citizens. And so, with the proliferation of stories in the media of funding restraints, hospital bed closures, long patient waiting lists, and government/hospital/physician power struggles, comes a growing sense of alarm.

While many health professionals, economists, and policy-makers emphasize that the time of plenty for health care is gone and that the situation will only become more desperate as this decade progresses, I am going to argue that, in fact, it can get better — a lot better — than it is right now. But this healing will not come about through the renewed flow of financial resources in some elusive future time, nor through technological breakthroughs in medicine, as impressive as these may be. The recovery of the health care system — and of the hospitals that are at its centre — depends on the better use of what we have right now.

This may sound to you a little like a cliché, the old "make do with what you have" argument. And of course, everyone agrees with the statement — but nothing changes. However, I am going to convince you that we can do more with what we have. The approach I will describe is the same as what the very best of today's businesses and industries, intent on survival and on energizing their successes into the next century, have created as the pathway to organizational transformation. It is called continuous quality improvement (CQI) or, more broadly, total quality management (TQM).

A comprehensive system of total quality management is proactive, a future-oriented strategy that will transform hospitals (and health care) from a crisis-management mentality to one of capitalizing on opportunity and leadership. The practice of total quality management — which emphasizes human skills, creativity and resourcefulness, customer satisfaction, employee involvement (or in today's vernacular, empowerment), effective and efficient use of resources, continuous improvement of all processes large or small, and the consistent achievement of high standards of service and productivity — can ensure that hospitals will maintain, and even increase, the quality of Canadian health care while slowly decreasing its share of the GNP.

For business and industry, TQM initiatives have proved difficult and many have failed. But for those that have succeeded in the total quality journey — such as Motorola, Xerox, and Federal Express — they are well positioned to ride out the rest of the recession and to flourish in the global economic restructuring taking place all around us.

In health care, TQM is relatively untried, and to many health institutions it's terrifying even to contemplate — because total quality management is far more than a tool for organizational survival. It is a visionary, dynamic process that leads not just to change, but to transformation. And transformation entails uncertainty, especially for those who work in hospitals. The bureaucratic structure of system upon system, typical of so many hospitals, is challenged and fundamentally altered by TQM.

In these pages, you will read the story primarily of how one Canadian hospital — St. Joseph's Health Centre in London, Ontario — shifted its patient care and entire organizational culture to an environment embodying total quality management. A few other hospitals — "quality pioneers" — have also begun the shift, and some of these you will encounter briefly.

What I am offering you is a snapshot in time of the effects of the transformative process of TQM at St. Joseph's Health Centre. It is the nature of TQM to change and evolve constantly, bringing into being new challenges and new realities. Even as I write, things are changing — new CQI teams have been launched, and improvements have been implemented, leading to the discovery of other improvement opportunities.

What is happening at St. Joseph's has already had a significant impact on the community at large. The January 1993 issue of *London Business Monthly Magazine* rated our hospital one of the ten best employers in the London region, citing the Health Centre's adoption of total quality management as an organization-wide philosophy and practice. "Of all the organizations participating in the 10-best survey, none came close to matching the number of essay replies received from St. Joseph's. It seems every employee has their own story to tell explaining why the hospital is such 'a great place to work,'" wrote journalists Janine Foster and Ken Maver. And a participant at a recent conference on total quality in health care in the U.S. observed that from his perspective the calibre of St. Joseph's total quality management initiative is equal to or better than the best U.S. health care organizations that offered presentations at the conference.

By continuously improving patient care and administrative processes and by recapturing much of the estimated 30 per cent of resources lost to waste and inefficiencies, total quality management in hospitals can help achieve the highest quality of service and patient care and make the best use of available health care system resources. But it takes time. Now that St. Joseph's has made that initial leap into TQM, the realization has dawned on administrators and staff alike that in our first two or three years into this process, we are only about a quarter along the way of what is, at minimum, a 10-year journey. Not until then can we claim for certain that TQM has fully permeated our organizational culture.

We *can* have better hospitals than we have now. We *can* serve our patients better. We *can* create high quality health care programs that reach thousands and thousands of people, even within the current climate of financial constraints. And even more excitingly, hospitals can bring this about *from within* their organizations. St. Joseph's physicians and staff have shown me and others how realistic this belief is.

We may reduce the size of hospitals. We may transfer some traditionally hospital-oriented programs to the community. But we cannot do *without* hospitals. When we are critically ill, when we need surgery, a life-saving medical intervention, or a complex treatment procedure performed by highly trained medical professionals, a hospital is where we need to be. And rather than waging a desperate uphill battle against escalating costs and rising public demand, hospitals can, in concert with the community, discover with total quality management a way to remain vibrant centres of healing well into the next century.

1

A Prescription for Change

From the changes I am prepared to make — that you are prepared to make — only then can we tell how much we really care about the Canadian health care system and each other.

— PHILIP HASSEN

For an entire year, Allan Tyson put his life literally on hold. Self-employed, in his mid-forties, and father of three, he could not make the decision whether to continue with his small, yet reasonably successful business, look for a less demanding job, or stop working altogether. He did not know if he should begin needed renovations on his home. He was not sure if he would be around for his daughter's high school graduation. Vacation plans were out of the question — even weekend plans. Indeed, he did not want to be more than a few feet from his telephone in case the call came through, the call that would start his life moving again. His overnight bag stood packed at the foot of his desk, at the ready for Allan to leave at any time for the hospital to undergo triple bypass heart surgery.

The major arteries to Allan's heart were seriously clogged, making him one of those patients for whom surgery was the best considered option, as opposed to those who could be better managed with medication. A chronic shortness of breath and a frightening, constricting pain that came on after only very mild exertion were the constants of his anxious days and long nights. The seemingly endless wait was an emotional rollercoaster; several times he had been given a date for his surgery at a large Canadian hospital, only to have it summarily cancelled.

Allan was only one of a long list of patients in his city who needed bypass surgery. As grave and debilitating as his condition was, it was not considered the most urgent. Five times he was bumped down the surgery list because another, more seriously ill, patient had priority.

"Every morning when I woke up I wondered if that day would be my last. Emotionally and physically I was in suspension — not dead, at least not yet, but not able to live either," Allan recalls. "The day my name finally *really* came up I was so elated, you would have thought I was being offered an all-expenses-paid vacation in the Bahamas rather than a hospital bed and a long uncomfortable period of recuperation.

"But at least I didn't end up as a newspaper story," he adds wryly, referring to articles he had read about patients with conditions similar to his who had died before they had ever got near an operating room. Such stories — of patients and their families squeezed between needed medical care and dwindling health care resources — raise a sense of alarm both in the public and among health care professionals, but seldom propose the possibility of there ever being a solution to the problem, or at the very least, significant improvements in the way health care is delivered despite the pressures to do more with less.

Almost daily, newspapers and television news broadcasts feature dramatic accounts of the critical state of Canadian health care — bed reductions, the closing down of entire floors in some hospitals, unreasonably long waiting lists for surgery and other specialized medical treatment, no money for important new programs, cutbacks in existing programs, angry physicians, overstressed health care staff, frustrated patients and their anxious families. Our hospitals' capacity to accommodate inpatients in acute care beds is being strained to the limit. And for the first time in many years, the economics of the 1990s has forced hospitals to lay off staff when the public demand for health services has never been greater.

Across Canada right now, health care is changing at a pace far more rapid and far-reaching than the system seems able to withstand. It would appear that the Canadian health care system, long the envy of many countries worldwide, is itself gravely ill. Some would even say fighting for its life.

To redress what has been considered an overemphasis on high-tech institutionalized health care and to attempt to contain spiralling costs, government health policy in this country is leaning more and more toward giving priority to the funding of community and home-based health services. The philosophical merits of this policy shift mean less disruption in people's personal and work lives, the delivery of care closer to home, less emphasis on high-tech medicine, and the strengthening of good primary care services through family practitioners and other health care personnel. But they do not allow for the fact that, even in ceding to community agencies the responsibility for certain types of health care — which perhaps hospitals should not have taken on in the first place — hospitals nevertheless must continue to play a central role at the heart of the health system. When we are critically ill, when we require major surgery, life-saving interventions, or a complex medical procedure performed by highly trained medical professionals, a hospital is where we need to be.

Canada's largest teaching hospitals today have budgets of hundreds of millions of dollars, amounts similar to, and in some case more than, that of many large corporations. Even the smaller community hospitals are dealing with budgets well into the millions. It is not surprising that, in commanding the lion's share of health care dollars, hospitals are currently under fire for their financial inefficiencies, service duplications, and bureaucratic obstacles to good management and delivery of care.

TOTAL QUALITY MANAGEMENT (TQM) AND
CONTINUOUS QUALITY IMPROVEMENT (CQI)

If hospitals have been identified as a large part of the health care system's problems, they must also equally become part of the solution. This urgently sought-for solution, as we approach the twenty-first century, cannot simply be more of the same. Strategies for effective delivery of health care services cannot focus on issues of controlling costs alone, as pressing as these issues are. The solution to what ails hospitals is, instead, to be found in new ways of managing, or more importantly, leading, hospitals and in the creation of a vision of hospitals' role to match new realities. The time has come for a radically different approach to running hospitals — the organization of patient care, medical education, research, outreach community care, hospital employee relations, administrative decision-making, and hospital board policy — an approach that emphasizes not cost control, but *total quality*.

Unless hospitals are prepared to undergo significant change in the way they are managed, no amount of number-crunching, cutbacks, or philosophizing will keep them viable. What is needed are not simply a few new policies or programs, but a fundamental shift in vision and practice that will transform hospital environments from today's crisis to tomorrow's opportunity. In the health care system of the future, hospitals must *lead* the way to real improvements, not simply react or valiantly struggle to cope.

Government has made it clear it will no longer bail hospitals out. Health institutions across the country are receiving the same blunt message: Do more with less; balance your budgets; eliminate your deficits; solve your own delivery of care and organizational problems. Our centres of healing — hospitals — are being told to heal themselves.

Media reports of the service cuts and layoffs, financial and organizational disarray, and patients dying before receiving needed treatment have done little to instil confidence that new ways of managing hospitals can result in health care that is more effective, efficient, and of higher quality than is currently the case. However, the sense of gloom that hovers over health care these days blinds us to potential new and effective avenues for solving the system's very serious problems and creating a more positive future for health care.

There *is*, however, a "prescription" for restoring the health of hospitals, both financially and in terms of the high standards of care expected by Canadian patients. But the origins of this prescription are not found in medicine, and its adoption by hospitals will bring about a radical new way of seeing, planning, and doing in health care. In business circles, it is called continuous *quality improvement* or, in a larger focus, *total quality management*.

TQM and CQI in Industry   An increasingly lean and competitive world marketplace has driven business and industry giants such as Xerox and 3M toward formulating and putting into practice strategies of total quality management. Customer satisfaction, cost benefit, employee involvement, effective and efficient use of resources, and ongoing commitment to quality are all seen as crucial to long-term business survival throughout the 1990s and beyond.

Since the mid-1980s, strong commitment to total quality has enabled a number of leading companies to turn million-dollar deficits into million-dollar profits, and others have sought the secret of their success. There is increasing conviction throughout the North American business community that in a difficult economy where downsizing, restructuring, labour unrest, and layoffs have affected even the most successful corporations, it will be total quality management, with its emphasis on human skills and resourcefulness and on the consistent achievement of high standards of quality in product, service, and performance — rather than an emphasis on costs — that will get business back on the road to economic health and productivity. We see examples of this today. Ford Motor Company, for example, has half as many employees today as it did in 1978, yet is producing almost the same number of cars.

Appropriately adapted to health care environments, these same concepts can support the continuing viability of hospitals in the present health care climate and as part of the economy as a whole. But because total quality management demands nothing less than a pervasive and far-reaching transformation of an organization, it is not an easy pathway or "quick fix."

In the business sector, while many high-ranking executives agree that companies can't afford *not* to adopt TQM, actually *achieving* it entails major risks; it means a dramatic shift in the organizational environment as traditional roles and the "this is the way we've always done it" mentality are challenged. Many companies have tried and failed. One survey of 500 U.S. manufacturing and service businesses found that only about one-third felt that total quality initiatives were having a "significant impact" on their overall competitiveness. Another study in Great Britain by the consulting firm A.T. Kearney of more than 100 British companies revealed that only one-fifth believed that quality strategies had achieved measurable results.[1] These less than spectacular findings caused many of the companies to wonder if total quality management was simply another fashionable yet ultimately dead-end management philosophy.

But Chris Green, a director of Ernst and Young's quality improvement consulting practice, believes that the reason for the failure of total quality management in certain organizations is not that a focus on quality is wrong, but that the implementation of quality was done either incorrectly or inadequately.[2] Green was commenting on the most recent in a series of reports of the International Quality Study conducted collaboratively by the American Quality Foundation and Ernst and Young on more than 500 companies in Germany, Japan, the U.S., and Canada, which found that total quality management initiatives did not appear to work for some organizations.

North American businesses and institutions, only at the beginnings of the "quality era," risk falling into the trap of trying to make unrealistic

improvements too fast. However, the evidence of many Japanese companies, which have practised total quality management for more than 40
years, and the impressive quality management successes of such major
North American–based companies as Motorola, Xerox, and Federal Express are strong evidence that quality management does achieve significant positive turnarounds.

Total quality management in an organization, whether in the private or
public sector, is not just an add-on human resources program or a matter
of training a few key individuals as quality "facilitators." In many organizations, the principles of total quality remain in the realm of talk and are
met with resistance from senior management and skepticism from front-
line workers. The authors of the British study found that in the companies
with quality programs that *did* succeed, responsibility for quality was given
directly to employees on the shop floor, the management structure had
been flattened, and functional barriers broken down.

TQM and CQI in Health Care Institutions   Hospitals experience many
obstacles — from the complexities of medical practice to "turfism" to
bureaucratic entrenchment to the sheer busyness of the hospital environment — in attempting to "walk the talk" of total quality. But of all possible
approaches to solving many of the health care system's problems, total
quality management, with its implications for patients, health professionals, and hospital administration, holds the most promise for achieving
long-term positive gains.

Managing a hospital is a complex and expensive undertaking, and the
money is running out. The minimal increases in funding currently being
allocated to hospitals by government in virtually every Canadian province
are fighting an uphill and seemingly hopeless battle with both rising costs
and the expectations of an increasingly knowledgeable and impatient
health consumer. (In Ontario, for example, hospitals received a mere one
per cent funding increase for 1992-93, and zero per cent increases for
1993-94 and 1994-95, which must accomodate any union contract settlements.) Forces in our current economic-political-social situation are
challenging not just the health care agenda of hospitals but, more importantly, the very basis and identity of our health care system. In attempting to sort out the complex interface between health care consumers, the
system responsible for the delivery of health care, and the role of hospitals
within that system, two facts are clear.

One, numerous opinion polls have shown that Canadians accord very high value to their health care system and will not accept any reduction in standards or accessibility. And two, health care costs have been escalating at such a pace they have now become unaffordable through public dollars. These cost problems could compromise the health system's accessibility and its standards of care. Further, the public wants more say in how their money is spent. This public expectation/cost dilemma faced by politicians, economists, health administrators, medical professionals — and patients — is not going to disappear. It is a fact of life for this decade and likely far into the next century. All health care stakeholders grapple with the urgency of the question: What will it take to maintain universal, equitable access to the publicly funded, publicly administered health care system in Canada today and tomorrow?

It is time for hospitals and other health care organizations to take total quality management seriously; it is time for them to utilize its strategies to transform their organizational systems and the delivery of patient care services. What happens economically and organizationally in health care has an impact not only upon hospitals and the patients they serve, but on business and economic health at the national and global level. Quality management of resources is no longer a matter of conceptual or philosophical debate. It is a necessity of practice.

Runaway health care costs may actually threaten Canada's ability to compete in world markets. Because health care costs drive product costs up generally, corporations may be even more tempted to bow to pressures to move production from Canada to the U.S. or Mexico. The fact that in Canada medical care is universally accessible with no up-front cost to the health care consumer has tended to obscure the crucial link between our standard of health care and the strength — or weakness — of our national economy.

In the U.S., total quality management has been making strong inroads with several major health care providers, such as Hospital Corporation of America, Intermountain Health Centre Inc., the Henry Ford Health Care System, and Kaiser Permanente. Donald Berwick's 1990 book, *Curing Health Care*, described the process and results of the National Demonstration Project, which in the late 1980s brought 21 health care organizations together with quality management experts from industry to explore how TQM methods could be adapted to the health care setting. Reporting on the hospitals, which achieved successful turnarounds by evaluating various aspects of their organization from a quality perspective, Berwick's conclusions are optimistic against the backdrop of the prevailing general despair about health care:

"We began it with hope, and we concluded it with confidence. We expected more than was reasonable, and we observed more than we expected. The efforts of these professionals, dedicated to excellence and asking only the chance to do their best, established a benchmark. We are confident that with time, resources, and committed leaders, quality improvement methods will flourish in health care as they have in other industries, and that all of us — patients, clinicians, managers, payers, and society at large — will profit."[3]

An example of one such positive gain Berwick reported was the improvement in discharging inpatients at the University of Michigan Hospitals. After analysing every aspect of what it takes to get patients discharged from hospital and back into their own homes, a multidisciplinary team consolidated preadmission procedures, admitting, utilization review, and the co-ordination of continuing care under one administrator. In this way, they could focus primarily on the causes of late discharge. Among the team's eventual recommendations were: improving communications concerning bed availability; including housekeeping staff in the communication chain; informing patients beforehand of transportation plans; developing a discharge planning process that would identify patients anticipated to have certain discharge problems; and having patient rooms cleaned at night to be ready the following day.

The result: Improved discharge planning reduced the average length of stay by 0.61 days for patients needing placement. Given the University of Michigan Hospitals' high occupancy rates, net savings were estimated at $250,000 a year. Quality discharge planning also had a positive ripple effect on admission procedures. Average waiting times after admission processing were reduced from an average of 3.1 hours to 21 minutes. During the period of July 1988 to July 1989, payroll and other costs were reduced by more than $260,000 a year.[4] Such is the potential of quality improvement processes — better service to patients and lower cost.

The challenges faced by the health institutions described in Berwick's book are considerable. The massive inefficiencies, ineffective systems, and inequities of the American health care system, inextricably bound up with a complex system of third-party insurance plans that nevertheless leave approximately 37 million Americans uninsured, have become a contentious and very urgent issue for the U.S. In 1990, U.S. health expenditures totalled more than $600 billion — 12 per cent of GNP. These costs are increasing by 13 per cent a year, twice that of other sectors of the American economy.

Whether or not the growing impetus from several quarters in the U.S. to reorganize American health care to incorporate some of the best aspects of the Canadian model gains ground in coming years, the commitment to total quality management by increasing numbers of American health care institutions signals a profound recognition that something different must be done. Massive health care expenditures cannot be allowed to continue unrestrained, even in the dynamic, market-driven, more *laissez faire* American economy.

In Canada, similar urgent concerns about the delivery of health care have a somewhat different context. Since the province of Saskatchewan pioneered publicly insured health care in the 1960s, leading to the subsequent adoption of universality in health care across the nation during the late 1960s and early 1970s, Canada is justifiably proud not only of the high standards of its health care system but of the right of all Canadians to have access to it. There are few elected officials in Canada who would propose to eliminate or significantly alter universal health care; for the Canadian public, medicare is an untouchable social value.

However, while it is evident that our policy-makers, health professionals, and the consumers of health care think highly of the existing health system and are loathe to consider changing it, many are also becoming increasingly concerned about the system's ability to cope in the present and meet the pressing health care needs of the future.

Canada has the most costly health care system of any other country with a nationally funded health service — more than, for example, Sweden, the United Kingdom, or New Zealand. Nine per cent of Canada's GNP is taken up by health care. In Ontario, the centre of much of Canada's key business and industry, the proportion of the provincial budget allocated to health care increased from 28 per cent to 33 per cent between 1980 and 1990. This percentage, representing one-third of the total provincial budget, translates into 1991-92 figures of $17 billion, of which almost $7.3 billion goes to hospitals.

It is nevertheless important to stress that total quality management, with its strategies of continuous quality improvement, as a pathway for hospitals is not just about controlling costs. In fact, one of the most common misconceptions of CQI strategies is that they are aimed primarily at cost containment. It is more a matter of realigning our present use of resources through streamlining what we do and asking whether what we do has any effect or achieves the intended outcome. In business, the consequences of correcting costly system ineffectiveness can run as high as 30 per cent of gross sales. But it is the commitment to quality, to doing the right thing right the first time, to focusing on customer satisfaction, high productivity, and excellent performance, that will ultimately drive costs down. The University of Michigan Hospitals' inpatient discharge team was concerned with streamlining discharge procedures to serve the needs of patients and enable hospital staff to do their jobs unobstructed by system inefficiencies — and in the process found that these service and organizational improvements also led to cost savings.

In other words, the achievement of quality most often leads to lower costs — a point missed by many businesses and public institutions which, with no clear goal in mind, are frantically chopping away at their high excess costs through mass layoffs and drastic service or production cuts. They are not viewing the situation from a quality perspective, which calls upon all stakeholders to play a role in creating a quality solution that will result in long-term win-win gains.

At first glance, the language of total quality management, which in the business or industrial sectors refers to customers and products, seems foreign to hospitals where phrases such as "patient care," "diagnosis," and "treatment outcomes" are the familiar terms. But by thinking as "customers" in the health care setting everyone who is served by the system — patients, physicians, staff, suppliers, and government — and by adapting "products" to mean the carrying out of all hospital procedures, hospitals will discover in TQM dynamic tools to enhance patient care, manage costs, and plan creatively for the future.

Total quality management in hospitals has to be designed specifically *for* hospitals. Implementation methods cannot simply be transplanted from industry or copied from another organization. Health professionals do not perceive their work as a manufacturing process. The use of such terms as "zero defects" is inappropriate for health care. Patients, unlike photocopiers or cars, are human beings with enormous individual differences in their treatment needs and health outcomes. Clinical outcomes in health care are tied to treatment plans that fit the needs of particular patients or improve the standard of care to groups of patients, rather than applying an identical treatment procedure in all cases.

Quality is providing the best possible care through continuously improving hospital services to meet the needs and expectations of patients, the physicians, the hospital staff, and the communities served by the hospital. It also involves making the best use of health care resources to meet those needs.

Continuous quality improvement (CQI) means that all hospital staff members are given the training resources, management support, and the time to become involved in constantly improving the systems in which they work so that they do their jobs better every day, providing the highest possible level of quality care.

Total quality management (TQM) is a systematic way of establishing processes and a structure that enable activities within the hospital to happen the way they are planned. It is a management strategy concerned with preventing problems from occurring by *transforming* the hospital into an environment where the attitudes and processes make prevention possible. The role of senior management — in demonstrating commitment, in giving leadership, and championing positive, hospital-wide change — is absolutely fundamental to getting a hospital on the quality path and keeping it there.

In order for total quality management to work in hospitals, it must take account of, and interact with, the current realities of modern health care — the economic, scientific, demographic, and social trends that are rapidly changing the face of medicine as we know it today and shaping the health care system of the next century, now only a few years away. Hospitals must also begin to understand and use the application of contemporary organizational knowledge.

THE CHANGING HEALTH CARE ENVIRONMENT

Most health care system analysts agree that the major threat to health care in Canada is rising costs, the fact that the capabilities of modern medicine are rapidly outstripping taxpayers' ability to pay for them. The relentless escalation of health care costs is being driven by a number of societal forces, each exerting powerful pressure upon funding resources, health administrators, and health care givers.

The rise in life expectancy and public expectation   Within this century, medicine has conquered numerous killer infectious diseases, such as diphtheria and polio, and has achieved control over chronic ones, such as diabetes or arthritis. We have better nutrition and higher standards of hygiene than our forebears, and our life expectancy has increased dramatically. As a society, we are healthier now than we have ever been.

Yet despite our overall good health and massive levels of government spending on health care in recent years, waiting lists for hospital beds continue to grow, and we wait longer and longer for elective surgery or to see specialists — even with a 60 per cent increase in the number of specialists over the past eight years — illustrated by Allan Tyson's situation described earlier in this chapter.

The fact of the matter is that the health care system is not one of supply and demand. Public expectation exerts enormous influence upon health care. Any significant increase in services, any new treatment procedures made available, will automatically create an excess in demand. For example, because organ transplantation has been developed as a viable treatment, patients who would benefit from this procedure will naturally want it. Raised expectations lead to raised costs.

But we are reaching a point where it is hard to justify constantly rising medical care expenditures with no end in sight. They certainly do not make economic sense, but to those who would argue that people's health is more important than economics, it can be shown that they don't make health sense either. There is no evidence to suggest, given the current high health status of Canadians (and of citizens in other developed countries), that more and more money spent on health care results in higher overall health or longer life expectancy.

For example, between 1960 and 1990 health costs as a percentage of GNP in Great Britain rose from approximately 4 per cent to 6.1 per cent. In Canada, the increase was from approximately 5.5 per cent to 9 per cent. Between Canada and Great Britain, there is a 2.9 per cent spread in the percentage of GNP spent on health care in 1990. We clearly spend more on health care than does Great Britain. But if we look at gains in life expectancy, we find they are similar for both Canada and Great Britain.

In 1988, life expectancy for Canadians was 73 for men and 79.7 for women. For the British, it was 72.4 for men, 78.1 for women. Between 1975 and 1985, Great Britain achieved a rise in longevity of 2.2 years. Canada achieved 2.85 years, about six months more than Great Britain. Therefore, the question is raised: Are those six months worth the many millions more dollars spent in Canada than in Great Britain?[5] Eventually, health funding in certain areas will reap diminishing returns.

Many public policy analysts also warn that runaway health care costs are eating into monies needed for other important programs — in education, the environment, justice, and social welfare — all of which are important to uphold and maintain the health of society as a whole. Strategies other than huge resource increases will have to be found to solve the problem of patients like Allan Tyson, and we will need to look to the evaluative tools inherent in a total quality focus for answers to make what we have go further.

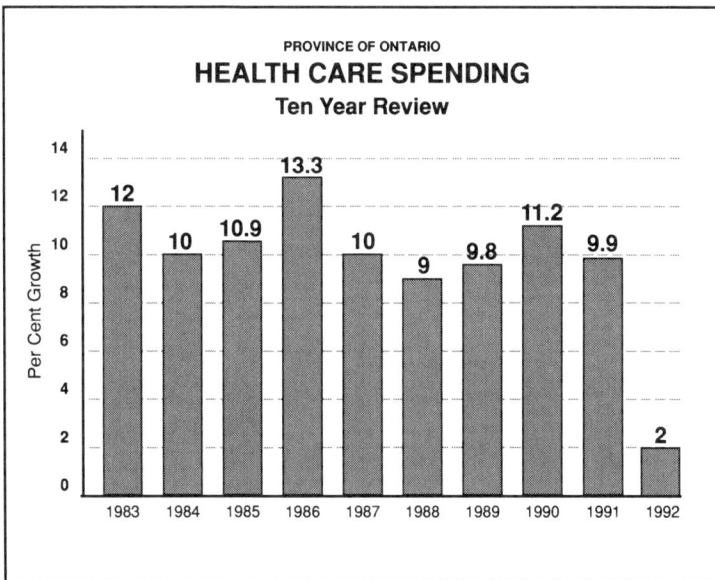

PROVINCE OF ONTARIO
HEALTH CARE SPENDING
Ten Year Review

Year	Per Cent Growth
1983	12
1984	10
1985	10.9
1986	13.3
1987	10
1988	9
1989	9.8
1990	11.2
1991	9.9
1992	2

The rise of technology   Powerful, sophisticated technology such as computerized tomography (CT) and magnetic resonance imaging (MRI), has revolutionized both diagnosis and treatment. On the positive side, the development of high-tech noninvasive diagnostic tests, as well as high-tech surgery and treatment, such as the use of lasers and fibre-optics, are important ways of making possible shorter hospital stays, less discomfort for patients, and more procedures being performed on an outpatient basis. The other side of the equation is that technology is extremely expensive. A CT machine costs about $1.5 million, an MRI machine $3 million.

The prohibitive costs of high-tech medicine, and its inappropriate use, are making it more and more difficult for any one hospital to contain all the technology it needs and wants within its walls. Increasingly, hospitals will be forced to co-ordinate and rationalize their technology-dependent diagnostic and treatment services among several institutions.

Technology raises other decision-making issues. Which technology should receive funding priority in future? Do we fund such high-tech "glamorous medicine" as organ transplantation or in-vitro fertilization, or do we focus on technology's role in delivering service in a wide variety of treatments, or better yet, effective prevention programs that reach more people?

Related to this is the need for evaluation of procedures both in terms of cost and effectiveness. New technology aimed at diagnosis or treatment is often put into place with no clear guidelines for evaluating whether its use makes a significant difference in patient outcomes. The development of such evaluation methods treads on the delicate area of physicians' use of resources — for example, regional surgery rates for identical procedures, or the appropriateness of ordering expensive diagnostic tests.

The impact of demographics   By the year 2021, 20 per cent of Canadians will be over 65. The need of older individuals for health services is often put forward as one reason for the rapidly rising health costs in Canada. But as studies point out, in many European countries, where the elderly make up an even greater percentage of the population, not as much is spent on health care.[6] Some analysts suggest that it is the number of high-tech "heroic medicine" services provided for the elderly at the end-stage of their lives, in many cases inappropriately, that exacerbate costs.

Nevertheless, the fact remains that older individuals are significant users of health care. Because we are living longer, the most common health disorders of the late twentieth century — heart disease, stroke, cancer, arthritis — require long-term management. The suffering and costs of Alzheimer's disease, which were not an issue at the turn of the century, are also part of the price we are paying for our longevity.

The demographic patterns of the young also affect health care. The generation following the baby boomers is not only much smaller in number, but today's young adults are marrying later and having fewer children. Down the road, this could well translate into a considerably smaller tax base available to support health care and other social programs. The impact of AIDS — in North America the prime killer of young adult males and insidiously making its way into the female population — is only beginning to be calculated in terms of its cost to health care and in terms of human devastation and death among people in their most productive years.

The shift to ambulatory, outpatient, and community-based care The capabilities of biomedical and instrumental technology have made increased outpatient and ambulatory care a viable reality. More patients can be served in an ambulatory setting, conceivably at lower cost, and with less disruption to their personal and work lives. However, one of the implications of this trend is that patients who must be admitted to hospital will be more critically ill. This situation will have an impact upon the stress levels of hospital staff, and upon hospital management and financial practices.

The delivery of care directly to people's homes through community agencies has become a public policy priority. In addition to the responsibilities for patient care within their walls — and, in the case of teaching hospitals, for medical education and research — acute care hospitals are being called upon as outreach resources for a wide variety of community-based programs. Long-term care hospitals are also being asked to forge even closer links with community agencies. While this shift is generally perceived as positive, there are many unanswered questions. How will increased home care affect the so-called sandwich generation, those who are raising children and carrying out career responsibilities, and who may also have to spend more time caring directly for elderly parents, no matter how much home care is available? And when the very frail elderly can no longer manage at home, what sort of institutional care will we offer them and how will we pay for it?

As well, what sort of prevention programs will best support a healthy old age? The medical director of St. Joseph's Centre for Activity and

Ageing, Dr. Peter Nichol, observes that much of the feebleness and lack of flexibility in old age is due to lack of fitness rather than organic illness. "I have had elderly patients who huff and puff and struggle just to get out of a chair. They don't have heart disease — it's that a sedentary lifestyle has left important muscle groups unused," says Dr. Nichol. "We have to get rid of this image that old age is a time for sitting around in rocking chairs; we have to get people moving."

Difficult decisions and ethical complexities The rationalization of hospital services is inevitable. In the future, there will be little, if any, government tolerance of duplication of services. Part of the task involved in implementing total quality management in hospitals will be the identification of a hospital's strongest areas of expertise and of the "customers" it serves best, and then the co-ordination of service with other hospitals based upon these characteristics.

In light of all the changes facing modern health care, difficult ethical issues come to the forefront. Rationalization may involve decisions as to which patients are eligible for procedures and which are not. Technology raises many sensitive and troubling questions, such as when to terminate life support systems, what constitutes informed consent, the limits of reproductive technology, and so forth. The medicine of the future is increasingly likely to be the "medicine of the gene." Advances in molecular biology and gene therapy, which have the potential to wipe out devastating human disorders, will also give rise to complex ethical questions.

All this, then, is the stage upon which hospitals today play out their medical, administrative, and human dramas. If, in the near future, these many difficult and costly issues are not addressed with energy, innovation, and commitment *within* hospitals, they will likely lead to draconian and radical cost-containment measures being imposed externally by government. When did government ever cut costs carefully while considering the quality of the results? In other words, it is up to hospitals, with their communities, to make themselves healthy, or else they will be forced to swallow some pretty bitter medicine.

THE ROOTS OF QUALITY

For hundreds of years skilled workers and artisans included inspection as part of the performance of their craft in the community. As the era of work performed by the individual skilled craftsperson waned and was replaced by factory-based shops, inspection became a management tool. Through the early influence of scientific management theorists, such as American Frederick Taylor, production eventually became standardized, and inspectors studied product samples using statistical methods designed to indicate the number of samples to be inspected and the criteria for acceptance or rejection. Interestingly, the basis of these statistical tools, now in the hands of workers, form part of the skills of CQI.

In the early 1930s, an influential book by Walter Shewhart entitled *The Economic Control of the Quality of Manufactured Product* questioned the effectiveness of product inspection. Shewhart claimed that problems in products were not as crucial as problems in the *processes* of work. Control of the process would lead to a better outcome than endpoint inspection.

But it wasn't until the aftermath of World War II that quality improvement developed into a fuller theory and practice. It was especially true in post-war Japan, which began struggling to regain an economic foothold in the global market. In the 1950s, the Japanese Union of Scientists and Engineers recruited one of the foremost proponents of quality in industry, W. Edwards Deming, whose groundbreaking ideas on the attainment of quality were being largely ignored in the U.S., to teach Japanese companies the use of statistical tools in solving quality problems.

Drawing upon the ideas of Deming and another American quality expert of the time, Joseph M. Juran, the Japanese began applying quality control to all aspects of production, including manufacturing, design, distribution, sales, and service. The combination of statistical techniques and the centuries-old group orientation of Japanese society, which emphasizes co-operation, respect, and collaboration rather than individual competitiveness, resulted in a powerful synergy of productivity and the achievement of overall high quality, which today is unmatched by other developed countries. As the Japanese began to design structures of management with both horizontal (across functions) and vertical (across hierarchal positions) impact, quality management expanded to encompass the entire workforce through the formation of "quality circles."

In *Curing Health Care* Donald Berwick notes that "many American companies slept through the early stages of the modern quality era. They failed to recognize the emerging competition in quality: competition based on improving customer satisfaction and reducing the costs of poor quality. Many companies collapsed, lost huge chunks of market share, or simply withdrew from global competition in many product lines."7

In the early 1970s, however, the quality circle concept began to permeate the American aerospace industry and subsequently spread to other industries. Another influence, besides global competitiveness, that paved the way for total quality management was the work on motivational behaviour by such theorists as David McClelland, Frederick Herzberg, Rensis Likert, and Douglas McGregor. Their insights informed some of the key tenets of continuous quality improvement: that people take pride in their work if they exercise autonomy over it; that recognition of creativity, innovativeness, and productivity creates a spiral of creative energy throughout the organization; and most important, that involvement, respect, and employees' ownership of their own work processes produce work of the highest quality with consequent high productivity.

How Quality has Been Managed in Health Care

Quality in health care is not foreign to hospitals, and the suggestion that Canadian hospitals must now make a shift to total quality management to remain viable and deliver high-quality health care does not imply that until now quality has never been a concern for hospitals. Health care professionals are dedicated to providing high quality services to patients, and all hospitals want to gain and maintain a reputation for high standards of care. But the management of quality in health care has traditionally followed the model of quality assurance (QA). Standards are set and individuals are held accountable by other individuals in the organizational hierarchy to ensure these standards are met. Moreover, standards are set by a department within the department itself and reviewed by its members. The structure is often arbitrarily set and frequently is not relevant to the services, products, or care delivered. Certifying, documenting, checking, and correcting are the central tenets of this approach. Solutions to quality problems are often framed in requests for increased resources, which in the current realities of health care are clearly unacceptable and probably should never have been acceptable. In today's health care climate, there are severe limitations to the effectiveness of a traditional QA approach.

Quality assurance does not enable a hospital to respond proactively to challenges and concerns about delivery of service. High-quality care can no longer be defined only as the achievement of standards. Quality has two features: quality in fact and quality in perception. Quality in fact results when the provider of a service meets understood specifications — the QA approach. Quality in perception is claimed only when customers believe their expectations have been met. Quality involves looking at the organization from the inside out, but also means evaluating ourselves from the outside in.

While QA focuses on standardized care and services within functions, most opportunities for improvement in hospitals actually cut across the organization and require a flexible, cross-functional approach. From the QA perspective, such opportunities are simply not apparent.

Little opportunity for employee involvement is provided with a QA approach; employees may be regarded as part of the problem. In today's health care environment, providers want to have a say in the improvement of the system. Furthermore, organizational research, particularly by Deming, has demonstrated that 85 per cent of organizational "problems" in the private sector lie in the "process" not "people."

THE CHARACTERISTICS OF TOTAL QUALITY MANAGEMENT.
Total quality management, appropriately applied in hospital settings, means providing the best possible care through continuously improving hospital service to meet or exceed the expectations of patients, physicians, staff, and the community. Total quality management requires the adoption, *across the hospital*, of several essential characteristics and principles. According to 3M Canada, the corporation that provided the base model for the development of an extensive total quality management initiative at St. Joseph's Health Centre in London, Ontario, there are five:

1. Quality is consistent conformance to customers' expectations.
2. Measurements of quality are through indicators of customer satisfaction, rather than indicators of self-gratification.
3. The objective is conformance to expectations 100 per cent of the time.
4. Quality is attained through prevention and specific improvement projects.
5. Management commitment leads the quality process.

These elements are the basis of a strong total quality management philosophy and through an implementation process that permeates the entire organization, are translated into behaviour that encourages, supports, and ultimately achieves quality. As mentioned previously, quality is attention to process but, more than anything else, depends on the goodwill, commitment, and enthusiasm of people who:

- are customer driven, both internally and externally
- develop the attitude that conformance to customers' expectations has top importance
- respect people and their ability to contribute to improvement
- understand that improvement includes everyone; in all parts of the organization
- place major emphasis on the prevention and problem-solving work
- involve employees in the decision-making process

Many would say that these precepts that guide the process are simple and self-evident, just the common sense of doing good business. Yet their simplicity is deceptive; actually implementing them is difficult. But it is worth both the time and the effort to take the risk of transforming Canada's hospitals using models of total quality. Of all possible alternatives being proposed to remedy the very serious resource and service problems plaguing our hospitals, total quality management holds the promise of being the most dynamic and progressive.

The chapters that follow elaborate on these precepts by describing in detail the development and implementation of total quality management at St. Joseph's Health Centre, a 960-bed teaching and research hospital. For total quality management to be successfully translated from the realm of theory to concrete practice in hospitals requires a sensitive balance between strategic interventions and human motivation. The organizational climate must be one that is ready both to receive and generate quality initiatives. The hospital has a substantial advantage if it is already functioning from a strong base of commitment to excellence — in the words of Theresa Marie Caillouette, General Superior of the Sisters of St. Joseph, referring to the century-old health care tradition of London's St. Joseph's Health Centre, "doing the ordinary thing extraordinarily well." Some experts in the quality field have observed that a key advantage for a hospital starting total quality management is that the majority of health professionals and health care employees have chosen their work out of a sense of service and a desire to help others.

Nevertheless, crucial to the success of TQM strategies, as well as the most significant predictor of whether a hospital can successfully adopt the quality prescription for better delivery of health care, is the human buy-in, the ability of all participants — patients, physicians, health care staff, administration, government, and members of the community at large — to understand and appreciate what's in it for them.

2

Beginning the Quality Journey

The fight for more resources is so familiar that it can feel naive and even dangerous to let go, even temporarily, of the battle, and to ask instead if a better process can be designed without more staff, more space, or more money — perhaps with even less. . . . More staff, more space, and more money almost never turn out to be the best remedies.
— DONALD BERWICK, *CURING HEALTH CARE*

Health care today revolves almost entirely around hospitals. Over the past two centuries, when such public health issues as hygiene, nutrition, and the prevention of infectious disease were resolved in the industrialized world, resulting in longer and healthier lifespans, hospitals became the prime setting for dealing with whatever serious illness *did* occur. And so we were led to believe we had solved our major organizational health care problems. We had generally healthy communities and a place for people to go when they were sick and needed specialized care.

THE END OF THE HOSPITALIZATION ERA
Much of the current stress and uncertainty in the health care system is that the "hospitalization era," as the dominant model for delivering health services, no longer meets the system's needs and demands. It is probably fair to say that when hospital systems were being developed, no one could have imagined the future costs of concentrating health care in hospitals. The outcome of this hospitalization era, which has evolved over many centuries, is that enormous amounts of money have been put into ensur-

ing that people with health problems are cared for in institutions. Over time, hospitals have rapidly become more complex, technologically sophisticated, and astronomically expensive.

The word "hospital" comes from the Latin *hospitalis*, meaning a "house for guests." In the Middle Ages, Christian religious orders were the impetus behind the founding of numerous hospitals whose mission was to care for the sick and the poor. The gradual decline of church influence in western Europe and the increased concentration of power in the state helped bring about the development of public hospitals. When, for example, Henry VIII abolished monasteries — many of which had hospitals — in Great Britain, the government was then forced to establish new hospitals. By the eighteenth century, public hospitals were the norm in Great Britain and hospitals modeled after the British institutions began to be built throughout Europe.

Today, both historical threads, the religious and the secular, are still found in hospitals. In most countries, hospitals are publicly funded and publicly administered, the notable exception being the United States where hospitals developed only partly through public initiative; private ownership has played a major role. Yet many hospitals originally founded by religious orders and churches still retain their spiritual heritage and values.

Discoveries by such nineteenth-century scientists and physicians as Louis Pasteur and Joseph Lister of how bacteria spread, the importance of antiseptics, and the potential of vaccination to prevent epidemics ushered in the beginnings of modern hospital care. These achievements, in addition to public health improvements in general, may be the most important factors in improving the overall health status of most of Western society today.

When it became possible to set up laboratories, organize clinics, and care for large numbers of patients in a safe hygienic setting, centralized hospital care seemed undoubtedly the most logical setting for physicians to conduct much of their medical practice. University faculties of medicine and hospitals saw great opportunities to establish major learning centres and research facilities to create new inroads for medicine.

The current crisis in health care — escalating costs with dwindling financial resources — delivers an inescapable message: *We have come to the end of the hospitalization era.* We cannot, in fact, must not, continue putting ever increasing amounts of resources into hospitals. Even if we had such unlimited financial resources, there is no strong evidence we would achieve the health gains for society we are looking for.

GIVING UP UNREALISTIC GOALS

American ethicist, Daniel Callahan, director of the renowned Hastings Institute in New York, suggests in his recent book on medical ethics, *What Kind of Life?*, that we ultimately want our health care system to defeat not just illness, but death itself. But if we want a reasonably affordable health system in future, we had better give up these illusions of immortality.

Indeed, some health economists have noted that the costs of delivering high-tech acute-care health services to the elderly are rising faster than any other health care cost. In many cases, the economists and some ethicists argue, we are not doing this to save lives or improve individuals' quality of life in their later years, but to prolong dying.[1] We need to do some serious thinking about what the concepts health, illness, quality of life, and treatment priorities realistically mean.

All this is not to suggest that hospitals will or should disappear. Indeed, their role in delivering an important component of current and future high-quality medical care has made them an indispensable part of the system. But as money has begun to run out, the most pressing issue is how to deliver the highest quality services with what we have rather than to bemoan what we cannot get.

Government, in its efforts to fashion new models of health care delivery, has begun making moves to "dehospitalize" health care with policy initiatives in the direction of community care. Hospitals themselves have been reducing their numbers of inpatients — downsizing — by initiating wide-ranging outpatient and ambulatory-care programs. These new directions, though generally viewed as positive developments, nevertheless have produced a sense of unease, even threat, within hospitals, by physicians and staff, and in the communities they serve.

Communities are attached to their hospitals, emotionally and economically. In many communities, the hospital is one of the largest, if not the largest employer. Thus when hospitals downsize, merge, dramatically rationalize their services, or in some cases are closed down, people get very upset. One TV newscast in early 1992 profiled the reactions of local residents to the possible loss of several small community hospitals in Saskatchewan. "We don't feel safe without our hospital," said one farmer. "The hospital is the heart of our community," said another, his voice shaking. And still another commented that even though it makes sense to try to save public money, it would be preferable to shut down the police detachment and move it to a neighbouring community than to close the small hospital.

THE NEED FOR A SEAMLESS SYSTEM

Future policy decisions are bound to fail if they do not address these questions: Is there a fundamental health service every community must have? How will locating hospitals mainly in larger centres, expected then to serve entire regions, combine with strategies of trying to deliver health care directly in communities? And what will be the long-term effects of economically driven decisions to cut services and close certain hospital facilities, decisions that in Canada, with its enormous land mass and widely scattered communities, disadvantage those in rural areas?

We cannot continue to view health care as a number of isolated systems — hospitals, community care agencies, public health, and so forth — that manage to get the job done, albeit with inefficiencies, overlaps, and sometimes very little communication among them. If our health care system is to deliver outcomes that actually serve individuals and communities as we understand it is to serve them, then the system must become seamless, an unbroken flow from community to hospital and, as appropriate, returned to community health and social service agencies as quickly as possible.

Saskatchewan has made a serious attempt to create such an integrated system. In Saskatoon and Regina Health Boards have been established to oversee the co-ordination of hospital and other health services. This involves the replacement of several hospital boards by the more com-prehensive Health Board and the mandate of Board Trustees to develop an overall community-based health care model of collaboration among hospitals and community health agencies. Similar strategies involving regional health care governance are being tried in New Brunswick. At best, these have been only tentatively accepted. Government-induced change has not yet been effectively adopted.

Whether such changes in the delivery of health care will be effective depends upon whether or not they provide concrete answers to crucial questions. For health care decision-makers, the focus must not be "How much can we cut or amalgamate and still survive?" but rather "Who are we serving and how can we continue to provide the high standards of care our health system has come to represent in the minds and hearts of Canadians? How can we determine that the services we provide are right, both in terms of appropriateness and outcome?"

THE INEVITABILITY OF SIGNIFICANT AND LONG-TERM CHANGE

It is in relation to these dilemmas that the concept of total quality management, with its emphasis on the importance of cross-functional teams in the delivery of service, shared decision-making, and continuous improvement, offers a potentially transformative direction for health care. We will have to deal with priorities. Which health services will receive public funding and which will not? Which hospital will provide what treatment? Which communities will have hospitals? These questions will require some fundamental rethinking not only of how we see these priorities but of how the system is to be set up. In the U.S., the state of Oregon has recently been a dramatic example of this complex — and conflictual — grappling with the issue of health care priorities and public funding by proposing a priority list of those procedures that would be funded for individuals receiving public aid and those that would not.

Since hospitals are being hardest hit with resource restraints in the form of smaller budget allotments from government and are being told in no uncertain terms to clean up their acts, the quality focus in health care must begin with hospitals. Precisely because they do still play such a central role in modern health care, hospitals are in the ideal position to be authors of significant change in the system if they so desire. They must *own* the future. If they are not able themselves to find strategies that successfully align economic reality, public expectation, and high-quality care, the reduction in the amount of available dollars will *force* change upon them — usually in the form of service cuts, bed closures, longer patient waiting lists, and increased government intervention.

Indeed, the one certainty about our health system is that there will be change far greater than most of us could have imagined. The way we do health care today will not work tomorrow. It is up to us as a society, and to those of us who administer health care and who deliver health services, to decide whether we continue on the old path toward the deterioration and ultimate dead end of a once dynamic system, or whether we strike out on a new pathway, taking with us the best of what we now have and making it better.

STARTING CHANGES BEFORE WE HAVE ANSWERS

Futurist Joel Barker, who has written extensively on the dramatic societal and organizational changes of the past few decades, has identified the qualities in individuals and organizations that allow work to get done: pattern-seeking, pattern-recognizing, and pattern-practising. Human beings naturally seek out patterns in their day-to-day lives and learn to use many of these automatically and unconsciously. You would not, for instance, want to have to relearn how to drive a car every time you got behind the wheel. If you are studying mechanical engineering at university or college, you expect the curriculum to be ordered in a certain way and to cover certain information. Patterns eventually evolve into rules and norms, ways of doing things, many of which are unwritten and also tend to remain unexamined and unchallenged — until they no longer work.

Much of Barker's work involves intense discussions within industry, business, and the public service sector concerning the "paradigm shift" propelling us rapidly into the next century. The phrases "old paradigm," "new paradigm," and "paradigm shift" have become rather popular jargon with business writers and organizational consultants. "Paradigm" is a word most suited to scientific and academic circles. Ask most people you know to define it, and chances are they will not be able to come up with a clear definition.

Part of the difficulty involved in introducing total quality management concepts into health care is that the language of quality and of paradigm change evolved in a business or industrial setting. In health care environments, these concepts must be translated into health care terms and the jargony buzzwords downplayed if total quality management is to have credibility with health care professionals.

The word "paradigm" is a lofty-sounding word for something rather simple, and is a useful concept for organizations, as well as individuals, seeking change. Barker defines it as "any set of rules and regulations (and they don't have to be written down) that establish boundaries and tell you how to behave inside the boundaries so that you can be judged successful."[2] In other words, it's the rules of the game.

When the rules change but you keep playing by the old rules, you eventually lose the game. An example Barker likes to share in his public presentations is what happened to the Swiss watchmaking industry. For centuries the Swiss were thought of as the world's supreme makers of watches and clocks. But when a bold and unknown inventor first tried to show Swiss watchmakers the enormous potential of the quartz crystal to replace the traditional watch mainspring, he was virtually ignored.

There were others who did take notice. Some years later, the Japanese announced a revolutionary new development in watchmaking — the quartz watch. As quartz timepieces caught on worldwide, the Swiss watchmaking industry was almost totally eclipsed, relegated to playing a minor role in the industry where it once had been a giant. Other examples of paradigm shifts are the change from manual and electric typewriters to desktop and portable computers, or from surgery using a scalpel to surgery using a laser. These are technical paradigm shifts. What we need are more basic shifts in our thinking and behaviours as leaders and providers.

Yet the attitudes and practices of the past are remarkably persistent, ingrained in our all too human tendency to be creatures of habit. "When people say, 'That's just the way we do it around here,' their paradigm has become unchallengeable dogma," observes Barker.3 And in today's changing marketplace, that is a prescription for failure. There is virtually no area of life today where the rules have not changed — family life, education, the workplace, leisure patterns, health care. What 1950s' radiologist could ever have conceived that the shadowy image on an X-ray plate would one day become a three-dimensional moving picture through the development of Magnetic Resonance Imaging, a technological breakthrough that has revolutionized the field of medical diagnosis?

Joel Barker is only one of an increasing number of voices beginning to articulate the idea that the total quality movement can both respond to and bring about the paradigm shift required for the rest of this decade and well into the twenty-first century. But most of us fear change, particularly when it means learning to carry out daily work in hospitals or anywhere else in a very different way from what we were first taught. As pattern-seekers, pattern-recognizers, and pattern-practicers, we want workplaces and our world to be predictable and stable.

Recent developments near and far bring home to us just how fragile predictability and stability are. The Berlin Wall is gone; the Soviet Union is no more. New nation states have come into being — some peacefully, some through war and bloodshed. The seemingly endless internal warfare plaguing modern-day Lebanon has all but erased the memory that this tiny country was once thought of as a Middle Eastern paradise.

The 1992 environmental summit in Rio de Janeiro, the struggle within

Europe to achieve a viable economic European Community, and the North American Free Trade Agreement are indicators that economic policies and social and environmental agendas, are no longer the concerns only of individual nation states, but have become major global issues. Across North America, thousands of jobs in the manufacturing sector have disappeared, the retail industry is in trouble, social programs are strained to the limit, and the gap between rich and poor widens.

Hospitals, then, if they want to begin a journey into the realm of total quality management, must take up the challenge of being paradigm pioneers in the face of much uncertainty and fear in the wider society. There is a risk, warns Barker, because "you can never prove that it will work before you do it."[4]

Total quality management in the first instance as a pathway for hospitals to assure the delivery of excellent health care within current resource constraints opens a whole new agenda for health care. It raises the question of how a health care organization with a total quality focus will behave, what role it will play in the health care system of the future, how it will be governed, who will practise within its walls, and how it will reach the communities it serves.

TOTAL QUALITY MANAGEMENT IN HOSPITALS IS IN ITS INFANCY
The concepts and practices of total quality management have really only had an impact on business and industry since the 1970s. For every quality success story in corporations such as Motorola or Xerox, there are three of failure. And once an organization has tried and failed, it has likely made itself resistant to total quality management for years to come.

The possible implications of total quality management for hospitals were first looked at by health care administrators and decision-makers in the mid-1980s. The first winner of the U.S.-based Healthcare Forum/Witt Award "Commitment to Quality" was the Alliant Health System in Louisville, Kentucky, in 1988; the Methodist Hospital System in Houston, Texas, won in 1989; the University of Michigan Hospitals in 1990; Intermountain Health Care Inc., Utah, in 1991; and Orlando's Florida Hospital in 1992.

Noting the changing attitude of North American hospitals toward establishing total quality programs, the 1991 International Quality Study (IQS) Health Care Industry Report, a study conducted by Ernst and Young and the American Quality Foundation of more than 500 acute-care hospitals in the U.S., Canada, Germany, and Japan, found that three years prior to its publication of data,

> less than 15 per cent of North American hospitals believed that the quality solution was to either "build it in" . . . or to "design it in." Today, those views are accepted by significantly more hospitals and are expected to be held by two-thirds of Canadian and U.S. hospitals in three years . . . Three years ago, a 'fix it in' approach — in other words, correcting service errors after the fact — was the primary philosophy of a third of Canadian hospitals and a quarter of those in the United States. That approach now has favour with 22 per cent and 23 per cent respectively of those hospitals, and its acceptance is projected to decline further. (However, it should be noted that the IQS found that the "fix quality in" attitude is still more prevalent in North American hospitals than it is within the banking, computer, and automotive industries.)[5]

Another finding dealt with the prevalence of simplifying hospital pro-cesses, one of the key objectives of continuous quality improvement. Only 6 per cent of American hospitals and as few Canadian hospitals reported they "always or almost always" apply process simplification practices — which means that patients and staff encounter a lot more hassles in hospitals than necessary. However, the hospitals saw the use of this process increasing to 40 per cent of hospitals within three years.[6] While in the business and manufacturing sector, the move toward continuous quality improvement is driven by the need to produce high-quality products and services in a globally competitive marketplace, the report sees hospitals' emerging interest in quality as influenced by "the demands of increasingly knowledgeable customers and a desire to control costs yet provide quality care."[7]

If the International Quality Study is accurate in its assessment of the number of hospitals intent on implementing quality strategies, and if the proliferation of conferences, seminars, and magazine and professional journal articles on quality in health care across North America is any indication, many hospitals are looking at the potential of total quality management for their own organizational culture.

One of the questions hospital administrators most often ask me — and I am certain the same question is asked of others whose hospitals have begun implementing total quality management — is: How did you get started? While there is no one way to start — each hospital's quality strategy must necessarily differ according to its organizational culture, size, and the communities of patients it serves — there are enough common factors that make sharing each other's experiences worthwhile. In the remainder of this chapter I will lay out the early initiatives St. Joseph's Health Centre took to create a culture receptive to the concepts of total quality management.

WHAT I'D LEARNED BEFORE COMING TO ST. JOSEPH'S

To put the St. Joseph's Health Centre's quality story into context, I will take you back to the early 1980s when I was executive vice-president of Foothills Provincial General Hospital in Calgary. Throughout my administrative career, I have always held a strong belief in the inherent connectedness of the workplace, that individuals work most effectively and experience the most satisfaction when they feel part of the whole organization.

However, in many workplaces, staff receive much rhetoric but little credible support concerning participation. Getting people involved in their work and giving them a say in the control of the workplace requires a different type of management from the traditional authoritarian and hierarchical structures we have grown used to in organizations.

I began to explore some of these ideas during my years at Foothills by embarking with key employees on a Quality of Work Life program in 1981. This program, which led to the creation of a Quality of Work Life (QWL) steering committee, was aimed at creating more positive union-management relations and at strengthening the willingness and ability of people to make choices in their work — the potential for individuals and groups of employees to influence the atmosphere, the environment, and decisions about their workplace.

One of the early Foothills QWL projects involved food services. As anyone who works in a hospital or has been a patient knows the jokes about hospital food often have strong basis in truth. Hospital food services are frequently the focus of customer complaints. Foothills' QWL steering committee met to review all aspects of food services, including doing a survey of patients and staff. Food services provided to staff were modified to be more appealing — for example, we created an outdoor café — and the committee looked closely at the food provided to patients, using "taste panels" to conduct evaluations. Because the cafeteria atmosphere was not considered very relaxing, it was renovated to become more aesthetically pleasing and conducive to staff needs.

Gradually more areas of the hospital were reviewed, operating on the principle that the people most qualified to solve problems with work are the people doing the work. For management, the focus began to shift toward managing systems rather than individuals, since individuals can manage their work more effectively without interference. This assumes the work goals are clear.

As the process of improving the quality of work life developed at Foothills, we then went on to create quality circles. It was around this time that the western world in general was hearing more and more about Japanese management — the participatory, noncompetitive style of management that has rocketed Japan from its reputation as a maker of junk to the producer of state-of-the-art quality in its manufacturing and service sectors.

At Foothills, we defined a quality circle as a small group of employees from the same work area who met regularly and voluntarily to identify workplace problems and implement solutions. Circles were established in such areas as health records, laboratories, physical medicine, respiratory medicine, the surgical nursing unit, the medical nursing unit, radiology, admitting, housekeeping, emergency, and the physical plant.

Quality of work life strategies, including quality circles, can, I believe, give hospital administrators and medical staff an intuitive feel for the possibility of further change that can be accomplished by expanding quality of work life into the wider context of total quality management. Total quality management is, in fact, a natural extension of quality of work life. Rather than focusing specifically on the workplace, total quality management encompasses all systems and processes of the entire hospital.

In the mid-1980s the Canadian public began to hear more about hospital deficits, along with warnings about the necessity of allocating resources and cutting some services to come to terms with tougher economic times. Until recently government was saying, "No more money," but nevertheless kept funding deficits. Hospitals and governments were equally at fault for the inadequate method of reimbursing hospitals for real work/care done. All hospitals were confronted with the challenge of how to continue providing the highest quality care at the lowest possible cost.

Around the same time, Foothills embarked on another important initiative, and this, too, laid the groundwork for a further evolution toward total quality management. Recognizing the need to do something concrete about the allocation of resources, Foothills, with the support of the Alberta Department of Hospitals and Medical Care, initiated a value improvement program (VIP), a strategy developed in the U.S. by the Baxter Foundation and implemented at Foothills and five other Canadian teaching hospitals.

At the heart of VIP are two requirements: the willingness to assess and evaluate internal costs and the practices behind those costs; and the ability to involve those who can affect changes in patient care. Comparisons to other hospitals are used to assist in the review of costs and practices. These comparisons probe deeply not only into dollars spent but into how physicians conduct their practices or variances in practice within hospitals, and into the implications of the hospital's own procedures behind the costs. However, the key factor is *quality*, not the compromising of patient care to achieve the lowest cost. At all times, the considered decisions of physicians and clinical staff determine actions appropriate for the individual hospital and its patient population.

Some of the first value improvement programs at Foothills included total hip replacement, myocardial infarction (heart attack), gall bladder surgery, cataract surgery, and materials management. Looking at the myocardial infarction (MI) task force for the period of November 1985 to April 1986, for example, two key recommendations had a major impact on patient care — the conversion of eight additional telemetry monitoring beds on the cardiology ward and the development of a system to identify low-risk patients. For simple cases — that is, patients meeting the low-risk criteria — total length of stay, which included time in the coronary care unit (CCU) and on the cardiology ward, dropped from 10.8 days to 6.7. For more complex patient cases, the length of stay in the CCU dropped from 7.3 days to 4.2, and 6 days on the cardiology ward fell to its target of 5.7 days; overall, the length of hospital stay for complex MI patients dropped by four days. These reductions represented a more clinically sound, efficient, less stressful hospitalization for patients but also significant cost savings. It was estimated that as much $300,000 annually was saved, which more than offset the initial $77,800 outlay for the telemetry monitoring beds.

Similarly, the value improvement program involving total hip replacement resulted in length-of-stay reductions of almost a week — 21.3 days to 14.6. Today, these lengths of stay are lower, but the important point is that the process created a change in thinking that continues to this day. By 1987, when the cataract-surgery study was added to the VIP initiatives, Foothills was able to report success in streamlined diagnostic procedures, revised medical practice, the development of new preadmission and discharge procedures, and systems for targeting low-risk patients — changes early on in the entire VIP process that effectively freed up the equivalent of 17 hospital beds and saved the hospital more than $1.3 million a year.[8] In 1987, Foothills was faced with reducing its budget by several million dollars. It did this by closing beds and reducing lengths of stay by more than a day per patient (from nine to less than eight), thus maintaining the volume of services.

Value improvement programs can be key tools for total quality management in hospitals, and I will say more later about how VIPs are designed and their role in helping to initiate total quality at St. Joseph's Health Centre.

EARLY STEPS AT ST. JOSEPH'S HEALTH CENTRE
As I look at my career to date, the shift in leadership philosophy and administrative practice that total quality management entails has been the most far-reaching personal and professional challenge I have ever encountered. I compare it to the time in young adulthood when I once left university studies and embarked on an intense inner search for the direction I wanted my life to take. As an administrative leader, taking on total quality management, I am challenged to question virtually all my pet assumptions. This is even more the case when the chosen setting for TQM is health care, rather than business or industry. In 1988, just before assuming the position as president and CEO of St. Joseph's Health Centre I attended a conference in Florida that was pivotal in developing new thinking about the evolution of quality of work life, quality circles, and value improvement. Entitled "The Critical Link," the conference, sponsored by the U.S.-based Healthcare Forum, dealt with the major changes taking place in certain key American businesses and industries involved in the concepts and practices of total quality management.

Many examples of quality successes in business and industry were shared at the conference, but there were also individuals who had come to explore the possibilities of total quality management in health care.

Donald Berwick, who now has the reputation as the "father" of the health care quality movement in the U.S., and another health care quality expert, A. Blanton Godfrey, were among that conference's participants.

The following year, another Healthcare Forum conference, "The Power of Quality," in California, was one of the first to begin dealing with the enormous potential of total quality management to create proactive strategies for dealing with an increasingly complex and financially troubled health care system. Several hospitals, some of which were participants in the National Demonstration Project on quality — which formed the focus of Berwick's book *Curing Health Care* — began reporting their experiences and some powerful results.

I attended "The Power of Quality" just after my arrival at St. Joseph's Health Centre. The conference simply deepened my growing conviction that total quality management was a visionary, transformative pathway for hospitals — and one that was possible. I began urging some of St. Joseph's senior management to attend similar conferences and seminars dealing with quality improvement in health care so that they, too, would get a feel for total quality management and how it might work at St. Joseph's.

One of the most important factors, and one I cannot stress enough, is that the initial leadership must come from the hospital CEO, senior management, and the board of directors. Without their commitment, total quality management will not work. Eventually quality will come to depend on many others, as well. But it begins with key individuals taking an interest, discovering its potential benefits, and then making decisions to act.

Gathering a team of individuals receptive to creating a culture of total quality management is, in my view, a key step very early on. Quality initiatives that will have significant and measurable success in hospitals cannot be introduced without a lengthy and careful preparation period — in St. Joseph's experience up to two years — in order to sensitize and refocus the hospital culture, identify its strengths and weaknesses, and find pathways for positive change.

Early in my tenure, the senior management structure was altered to eliminate two layers of management — the position of chief operating officer and other senior management positions — to begin creating the flatter, less bureaucratic structures management experts were saying, and I believed, would characterize the most successful businesses of the future.

Introducing the concepts of total quality management must go well beyond senior management, however. There must be a critical mass of people within a hospital motivated and committed to total quality management. You will never get past the early stages if the organization cannot internalize the philosophy and practice of total quality. With this in mind, we began to involve not only senior management, but other managers who were deemed initiators or risk-takers. We invited several noted speakers to address them; an organizational consultant did a presentation on the importance of understanding organizational culture; another conducted a one-day seminar on the agenda of quality; and managers began to read relevant articles and books, such as Tom Peters's *Thriving on Chaos*.

Hospital-Industry Collaboration   As St. Joseph's Health Centre began its search for possible models of quality management, a golden opportunity presented itself from our hospital board room. John O'Neill, now a vice-president at 3M Canada, was at that time chairman of the board for St. Joseph's. In the late 1970s, 3M had begun extensive research into the "managing total quality" process, and through the 1980s emerged as a leader in implementing total quality management strategies throughout the corporation. Because of its early and successful involvement with total quality management and its being a major supplier of more than 5,000 products to the health care industry, 3M was interested in helping to ensure the continued strength of health care.

In early 1990, St. Joseph's Health Centre and 3M began the collaboration that would allow the Health Centre to adapt 3M's extensive materials to fit a Canadian hospital environment. The St. Joseph's Health Centre/3M collaboration was one of the first in Canadian health care; there are now several other hospitals beginning to use 3M materials, among them Women's College Hospital in Toronto.

The presence of John O'Neill on the Health Centre's board was instrumental in the match between 3M's quality expertise and St. Joseph's quality vision. This is a point particularly worth noting — that quality models and their teaching tools may indeed be available to quite a number of hospitals. Most hospital boards have representatives from the business and industry sectors among their membership. Some of these individuals may be working in companies that have taken significant strides toward total quality management. There is the potential for a wide variety of innovative industry/health care quality improvement collaborations across Canada. Since 9 per cent of Canada's GNP is spent on health care and, if present trends continue, this figure will rise, it behooves the business and industry sectors to take an active interest in the potential of quality management to affect health care costs.

St. Joseph's Health Centre had also begun some early attempts to use the concepts of customer focus and value improvement programs on a number of projects. A value improvement program was set up in the area of obstetrics — looking at normal labour and delivery; and one in the area of surgery — evaluating routine gallbladder operations. Both were set up in a similar vein to those at Foothills Hospital. And an important new patient program — the Western Ontario Provincial Lithotripsy Program — was designed from the start with a customer (patient) focus, and provided some early evidence that this focus results in cost-effective outcomes.

For example, Peter, a 56-year-old London resident, suffered from recurring kidney stones for several years. Up until 1990, he would have been referred to Buffalo or Toronto for lithotripsy, a high-tech, non-invasive procedure that breaks up kidney stones by means of high-energy shock waves. He would have been on a waiting list for several months.

Before lithotripsy, which first became available about eight years ago, Peter would have had to undergo surgery requiring a stay of up to 10 days in hospital and six weeks of recovery time at home. The cost to the hospital would have been about $6,200. But if Peter had a kidney-stone attack tomorrow, he would remain in southwestern Ontario and be immediately referred to the lithotripsy program established by Dr. John Denstedt at St. Joseph's Health Centre in August 1990. He would be treated as an outpatient and be in and out of hospital in four or five hours. He would return to work in just three or four days. And instead of $6,200, St. Joseph's lithotripsy program cost about $900 a patient in 1990, about 33 per cent less than the same service at another Canadian hospital. Today, this procedure costs less than $650, a real tribute to the staff and physicians involved.

Granted, advances in high technology, of which lithotripsy is a dramatic example, allow for more procedures to be performed on an outpatient basis. But the patient-centred processes tailored specifically to St. Joseph's lithotripsy program, rather than simply copied from a problem-solving model, account for much of the savings. These improvements include a highly effective way of scheduling patients that includes preadmission lab work, and a streamlined, well-organized co-ordination among all involved departments. I've included more about the customer-centred design of lithotripsy services in Chapter Three.

Buoyed by these early clinical successes, the commitment to continuous quality improvement at the Health Centre intensified, particularly among physicians and other care givers. One of the Health Centre's senior obstetricians, who was an integral part of the labour-delivery study team, observed that the opportunity to evaluate every aspect of the process, from admission to discharge, was a valuable and instructive exercise. "Every physician should have this experience at least once," he concludes.

In May, 1991, senior management participated in a three-day retreat where the focus of the workshops was on beginning to understand and apply the concepts of total quality management. The Health Centre also made a commitment to hire a director of total quality management, a position new to health care but crucial to the long-term success of total quality management in a hospital environment. The role of the director would be to facilitate the acceptance of change across the hospital as it evolved toward a culture embracing total quality management. And a major impetus was our success in obtaining a $300,000 Ontario government grant in mid-1991 under the Health Innovations program of the Premier's Council on Health, Well-Being, and Social Justice.

Another move that senior management felt was crucial was to involve the hospital board in the very early stages. Beyond the fact that a hospital board member was instrumental in helping to bring about the collaboration with 3M, quality began to be discussed as a regular feature on the board's agenda. When the board worked on revising some of its bylaws, responsibility for quality at the Health Centre was made central to its overall mandate. Eventually the board established a pilot committee, the Patient Care Committee, and began to consider the issue "Who are our customers?" from a board perspective. As a result of the pilot, this group has been renamed the Quality Care Committee.

Health Centre senior management also spent time reviewing the key learnings of corporations with a track record of positive results from total quality management. These key learnings, included in the 3M training material, can be summarized briefly in eight points:

(1) **Continuous quality improvement requires change at every level. Change is difficult and must be managed.** Total quality is

built upon the reality of global economic and social change. People must learn to manage change so that it does not defeat the potential for a dynamic, positive future.

(2) **Management must lead and be totally involved.** You cannot delegate total quality management. Whether in a private corporation or a publicly funded institution such as a hospital, management must be visible and committed to the process.

(3) **Emphasize people.** People are the heart of total quality management. The quality improvement process involves determining peoples' expectations and meeting or exceeding them. This priority, emphasized *internally*, moves outward to the *external* customer (in the case of a hospital, patients and the community at large).

(4) **A specific process model cannot be transplanted.** Total quality management is created within an individual organization's culture. It cannot be transplanted from organization to organization. In particular, an industrial quality model cannot be transferred as is to health care, but must be carefully adapted.

(5) **The process is best facilitated by people from inside the organization.** If you want total quality management to permeate the entire hospital culture, hospital staff must be trained to implement every aspect of quality improvement. Most of the teaching of continuous quality improvement processes must be done internally, as well.

(6) **An annual plan must drive the improvement process forward.** Many hospitals are very adept at developing long-range strategic plans. But total quality management requires the inclusion of an *annual* plan that will focus the hospital on the achievement of its quality goals.

(7) **Follow-up becomes a predominant feature of the improvement process.** Review, revise and change become operative principles in a quality organization.

(8) **At the heart of quality is anticipating and meeting customers' needs, and exceeding their expectations.** In the case of hospitals, the patients and the communities served by the hospital are naturally understood to be the customers. But fundamental to total quality management, we must also serve internal customers — the hospital staff. Learning and meeting their expectations, too, will strengthen the hospital's overall quality focus in serving the end-users — the patients.

ESSENTIAL CHARACTERISTICS OF QUALITY IN HEALTH CARE

Without a commitment to the values underlying the quality process, total quality management in hospitals will be reduced to an activity-based program. Total quality management has the potential to dramatically alter hospitals as we know them today if it becomes a strategy that also looks into the mirror and faces the myriad of inept systems we have created. The principles of quality must be grasped first by those who must lead the process, and then must be thoroughly taught and understood throughout the hospital. St. Joseph's Health Centre's quality-training literature refers to these essential characteristics as the seed or "genetic code" of total quality management.

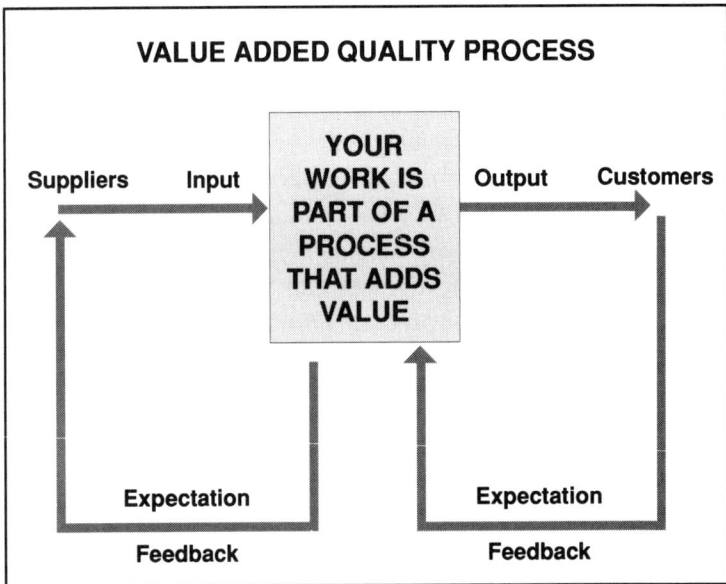

VALUE ADDED QUALITY PROCESS

Suppliers   Input   **YOUR WORK IS PART OF A PROCESS THAT ADDS VALUE**   Output   Customers

Expectation   Expectation

Feedback   Feedback

It is particularly helpful for hospital staff to understand the use of the word "customer" in relation to health care. Each person in a health care organization either gives or receives a service or product. The customer is anyone who receives the product of a health care organization's labour. External customers are people outside the hospital who use its services — patients, their families, universities and community colleges, government, and community physicians.

Physicians use hospital facilities and depend on the hospital to care for their patients. And in serving patients, hospitals also serve patients' families and patients' other support systems within the community. Educational institutions depend on hospitals to train health professionals. Government expects hospitals to use their resources well to maintain and improve a health system that is admired around the world.

Internal customers are understood as people inside hospitals who rely upon each other's services — nurses, laboratory personnel, researchers, clerical workers, kitchen staff, physicians, and so forth. Every person in the hospital is part of a continuous cycle of receiving service from an internal supplier and passing it on to yet another internal customer until the service reaches the end-user — the patients and their families.

The five essentials of quality, applied to health care, have one primary ultimate aim: to benefit the tax-paying consumer of health care — patients — who receive the medical expertise and attention promised and expected. St. Joseph's has expressed them as follows:

Essential #1: Quality Is Always Meeting Customer Needs and Exceeding Their Expectations Once health care organizations understand who their customers are, the next step is to consider what role customer expectations play in the achievement of quality health care. It is hard to define what quality is, but people certainly know when it is missing. All of us tend to judge quality by our impressions of whether or not we have received good service. If you're kept waiting in line for half an hour in a busy retail store, your annoyance will likely cause you to feel you have received poor service, no matter what the quality of the merchandise.

Likewise, if you are sent for a medical test, say a CT scan, and you are kept waiting for an hour, then are quickly put through the procedure with very little explanation of what to expect and no idea of when your physician will tell you the results, you'll probably be left feeling anxious or annoyed — regardless of the accuracy of the test and its provision of a basis for excellent clinical care. In other words, you did not get what you expect — which is courteous, caring treatment.

Often in the public sector the view has prevailed that the customer has no choice; you cannot normally shop for health care the way you do for a car or personal computer. When you need medical treatment, the hospitals and clinics in or near your community are generally where you will go. You might ask why, then, be concerned with the customer's expectations? After all, we should be grateful to have such a good publicly financed health system in the first place.

At the very foundation of the total quality movement in health care is the recognition that people deserve the best care possible. People who are ill, wounded, or disabled must for a time rely on the health care system for the help they need. Not only are there moral and humane values attached to health care, but we must also be mindful that patients are taxpayers and in a publicly financed system have a right to health care services.

As well, meeting customer expectations in health care has now become a matter of survival for health organizations. A health facility that repeatedly dissatisfies people loses not only professional credibility and community status, but perhaps the right to offer certain services, develop new programs, or even to remain in operation.

Essential #2: Use the Customer's Measure of Quality   In the new environment of total quality management, hospitals are asked to see everything they do through their customers' eyes. It may well have been the case that the CT scan administered to the anxious and annoyed patient was the right test, performed correctly, with equipment built and maintained according to standards.

But while conformance to standards is a step in the right direction, it is not enough. Defining quality as conformance to specification alone is a product- or service-oriented definition, not customer-oriented. If a hospital's service simply meets specifications that other facilities meet in basically the same manner, the hospital's service level has become generic. In these days of the rationalization of health services, the hospital that believes it is the best qualified to manage certain programs, or to deliver a unique, specialized program, must prove it can surpass the generic.

If there are two or more facilities in your city where people can go for day surgery, for example, on what basis do you choose one over the other? The facility that has clearly identified its customers and then takes steps not only to meet the expected standards shared by all facilities but to exceed the customers' expectations in terms of satisfaction, effectiveness, and efficiency is the hospital with the quality edge.

Essential #3: The Objective Is to Consistently Achieve Error-Free Work throughout the Organization   Errors in the operating room, wrong diagnoses, incorrect medications — these translate into the human cost of someone becoming disadvantaged, perhaps permanently, by the system he or she depended upon for help. For health care givers, errors or mix-ups translate into energy being drained from patient care through the added stress of dealing with constant system inefficiencies.

Mistakes and errors will rise to the level management will accept. If 15 errors a week are okay, then that is what you will get. If an organization is closed, geared to protecting the status quo, there will be no effective system in place to track down the causes of errors and initiate improvements. With total quality management, however, the hospital is constantly and consistently driven to achieve error-free work throughout the organization. The goal is not only to do it right, but to do the right thing right.

Essential #4: Quality Is Attained through Prevention and Specific Process-Improvement Projects   The most effective approach to being able to always meet customer expectations is error prevention, rather than simply error detection. The detection approach to quality is a great gamble, particularly in health care. Hospitals by their very nature are technologically complex and busy environments. There are risks enough without relying on a quality program that acts only after the fact.

Error prevention involves changes and improvements in the *system* developed and implemented by hospital management, and the design of new programs with a customer-centred, not problem-centred, focus. Input from staff must be sought to bring about changes and improvements in service processes and work procedures.

Essential #5: Management Leads the Quality Process   Senior management, with its total commitment, must lead the way. I cannot emphasize this enough, because the success of total quality management absolutely depends on it. The high failure rate of total quality management in organizations, identified by management analysts and researchers, is due in large part to lack of long-term management commitment or to the inability of management to communicate commitment in a credible way. Real management commitment entails concrete action resulting in real improvements, not good intentions expressed in empty words.

LEAPING FORWARD INTO "CRAZY TIME" —
CONFRONTING THE BARRIERS

In the transition to a model of total quality management, St. Joseph's Health Centre inevitably found itself in the midst of "crazy time," the tense period between the present and the future. There were, and still are, the uncertainties, unanswered questions, and discomforts that accompany any significant transformative change.

Change is scary. The management approaches that are central to total quality management threaten the older authoritarian, role-defined ways. A hospital intent on evolving toward total quality management must be prepared to live through this crazy time and still deliver the high standards of care expected by patients. This is the time when the barriers to total quality management will make their presence known, sometimes dramatically, often more subtly.

Many of these barriers we identified at the May 1991 management retreat. Some are common to all organizations undergoing change; some are unique to health care. With the help of a fishbone diagram, we outlined major barriers under six headings:

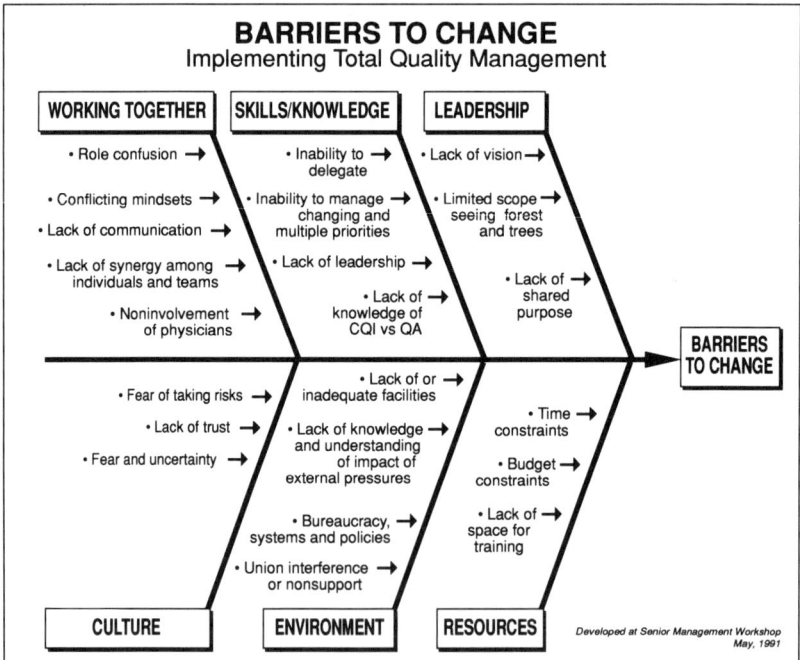

BARRIERS TO CHANGE
Implementing Total Quality Management

WORKING TOGETHER | SKILLS/KNOWLEDGE | LEADERSHIP

• Role confusion →
• Conflicting mindsets →
• Lack of communication →
• Lack of synergy among individuals and teams →
• Noninvolvement of physicians →

• Inability to delegate →
• Inability to manage changing and multiple priorities →
• Lack of leadership →
• Lack of knowledge of CQI vs QA →

• Lack of vision →
• Limited scope seeing forest and trees →
• Lack of shared purpose →

BARRIERS TO CHANGE

• Fear of taking risks →
• Lack of trust →
• Fear and uncertainty →

• Lack of or inadequate facilities →
• Lack of knowledge and understanding of impact of external pressures →
• Bureaucracy, systems and policies →
• Union interference or nonsupport →

• Time constraints →
• Budget constraints →
• Lack of space for training →

CULTURE | ENVIRONMENT | RESOURCES

Developed at Senior Management Workshop May, 1991

People working together When an organization starts shifting to total quality management there will be much confusion about roles, particularly management roles. At the centre of total quality management is a flatter, less hierarchical organization and an emphasis on self-directed and cross-functional teams. Managers, both senior and middle, are unsure of the implications of total quality management for the way in which they are to manage. People with rigid mind-sets will often feel the greatest sense of threat and offer the greatest resistance. Communication is also an important issue, since people will feel disenfranchised if they don't know what's going on and feel uncertain about the changes happening all around them.

Culture/Relationships Fear is by far the most crippling barrier to the success of organizational change. People want a sense of security in their workplaces which unfortunately in today's economic climate no longer exists. When hospital staff see colleagues at our or other hospitals being laid off or read about numerous industrial and business layoffs, there is understandable fear that the new direction of total quality management may mean job loss.

I stressed to staff from the beginning of St. Joseph's total quality management initiative that no one would lose his or her job as a result of the efforts toward total quality management. We have lived up to that commitment, energizing the confidence people have in what we are doing. No organization will successfully implement change if people feel personally at risk in making improvements. People must see the benefit of changing what it is they do at work for them and the organization to be successful. Our goal is to move people from the fear of transformation to the transformation of fear.9

Another aspect of the fear is related to the first category about people working together. Staff may not feel comfortable dealing in a more egalitarian way with managers and physicians, while managers may be uncomfortable with a more autonomous staff who expect to participate meaningfully in decision-making. Much work must be done to create a culture where people feel safe to raise questions, try new behaviours, and learn from mistakes.

Skills/Knowledge As staff learn new tools for continuous quality improvement, managers and other staff who still resonate to the old way find it difficult to delegate responsibility for the use of the tools. Strategies for continuous quality improvement also call for individuals to be able to manage multiple priorities. For some, the perception that it takes a great deal of time to fully understand and implement these strategies is a significant barrier.

Environment   Total quality management in health care will not succeed if health care providers don't have an understanding of the external pressures being brought to bear on the health care system as a whole. The reasons a hospital is implementing total quality management must include a realistic discussion of current health care system realities.

Another significant environmental barrier is the bureaucratic structure of many hospitals — indeed the large number of mini-bureaucracies and complicated systems that have been created in hospitals for getting things done. In some hospitals, such as ours where we have three main facilities — St. Joseph's acute-care building, the St. Mary's chronic-care facility, and Marian Villa (a home for the aged), as well as several off-site satellites — the complexity of the facility itself is a major barrier to setting up continuous quality improvement projects, but more particularly, to communicating them throughout the organization.

Traditionally, hospitals have been organized along departmental lines — clinical services, therapeutic services, laboratory and research departments, food services, and so forth. Solutions to problems and errors have also tended to happen on a departmental basis, with the result that any improvements achieved are often only partial. If you look at the process — from admission to discharge — by which patients are served, you find that many departments and many functions are involved. The way hospitals are organized into functional and professional groupings is often a barrier to effective service to patients, as well as to meeting the needs of hospital staff in their efforts to serve patients better.

Hospitals are no strangers to complex systems. In an attempt to deal with constant new developments in health care — whether medical or economic — we have created system upon system, but these have largely ignored the relationship of one departmental system plan with another. In other words, hospitals are often blind to the cross-functional nature of how health care is accomplished. It is not simply the realm of physicians or nurses. There are also the lab, the kitchen, porters, therapists, administrators, maintenance personnel, and numerous other individuals and processes. Peter Drucker, one of the authors of the ground-breaking books on organizational excellence that appeared in the early 1980s, has said that hospitals are the most complex organizations he has ever seen.

Under "environment" barriers, we also included union-management relations. Many hospitals are required to negotiate a number of collective agreements, and if the union-management relationship is adversarial, much of the potential for quality solutions to problems in health care will be lost. The situation, of course, does not only occur in the hospital setting. The model of union-management negotiations currently in much of business and industry is, in North America, strongly adversarial. There is a management agenda and a labour agenda, and each tries to muscle the other into a win-lose position. At St. Joseph's Health Centre, we realized very early on the importance of involving our unions closely in the total quality management planning process and to begin to forge partnerships, which while not always agreeing, are successful in attaining many win-win results (more of this in Chapter Six).

Leadership　Barriers to total quality can arise from the leadership itself. Total quality management requires first a clear and courageous vision of the future. It then requires leaders who can see the forest as well as the trees. It is not enough for senior leaders in an organization to *say* they are committed to total quality management; they must arrive at a common vision and a sense of shared purpose with the institutions they are serving. In Chapter Seven I will expand on this vital point. The good news and the bad news is that our future is very much in the hands of our leaders.

Resources　The major resource barrier to total quality in health care, as in many other busy organizational environments, is time. "Where am I going to find the time for all this?" is a refrain often heard at St. Joseph's Health Centre. Yes, a good deal of time *will* be required, particularly at the outset, but if this barrier is to be overcome, people must come to understand that eventually continuous quality improvement will be implicit in everything they do. It will have become *the way work gets done*. It will be a way that will help staff work smarter, not harder.

The other resource barrier many hospitals raise is money. There is a mind-set in health care that effective new programs need large amounts of money. While there is bound to be some cost in the initial phases, particularly if hospitals employ good outside consultants to help get the process started, the process can unfold from within by drawing upon the educational resources, talents, and flexibility within the organization. This has been demonstrated by those organizations in business, industry and health care that are beginning to see enormous success through this strategy.

PLACING OUR BETS ON TOTAL QUALITY MANAGEMENT

When the implications of the five essentials of quality are understood, it soon becomes evident that the shift to total quality management in our hospitals requires nothing less than a far-reaching paradigm shift, to use Joel Barker's phrase. New realities create new rules.

Right now in Canada there is strong government interest in the potential of total quality management for health institutions. One of the priorities of Ontario's deputy minister of health is the creation of a quality agenda for Ontario health care and this is no doubt the case in every Canadian province. Across the country, politicians, policy-makers, and most importantly, those in health care themselves are beginning to understand the importance of finding a better way for health care in the future. There are at least three significant examples of how important this movement is to major national health care organizations.

First, I could never have foreseen that the Canadian Medical Association would take on total quality management with such fervour as it has recently. The CMA has begun developing training and skills programs for physicians. This commitment is a vital indicator of the importance the CMA attaches to issues of total quality in health care.

The second example is the Canadian Hospital Association. The CHA is in the process of finalizing its vision statement for health care in the future and points to the need for the transformation of health care organizations of the future.

Third, the Canadian Council on Health Facilities Accreditation is trying to decide how far to lead hospitals into the quality movement's organizational transformations. The complexity of this dilemma revolves around whether the council's "standards" should lead the field of hospitals and health care agencies or whether it should follow them into the quality movement. My emphatic response is, *they should lead.*

At a time when it is not yet clear to us what this model of total quality in health care will look like, there nevertheless needs to be a sense of reliability and trust of the process fostered throughout the hospital and also with the public the hospital serves. I believe this begins first with the hospital CEO who must admit his or her own need to learn, change, and grow.

As I stressed earlier, total quality management is only in its infancy in Canadian hospitals. There are some U.S. hospitals who are further along, but they will be the first to tell you they still have a long way to go. At St. Joseph's Health Centre, I believe we have come far enough to have an exciting story to tell Canadians about the potential for transforming health care. I am willing to bet we will succeed.

3

The Physician's Role In Total Quality

Perhaps the most significant resistance to change comes from the fact that the leaders have to indict their own past decisions and behaviors to bring about change. . . . Psychologically it is very difficult for people to change when they were party to creating the problems they are trying to change.

NOEL TICHY

I don't have time for all this continuous quality improvement stuff the hospital's administration is getting into these days. I already serve on hospital committees," grumbled one hospital physician, glancing out his office door at a waiting room full of patients. "What about time for my patients? There are hundreds of them and I am only one person. And what about time for my research, not to mention a personal life? Management of the hospital is administration's job; mine is taking care of patients."

Physicians are the one group within health care to whom we will have to do an exemplary job of selling the idea of total quality management if we want to achieve our new vision of health care.

Total quality management as a transformative direction for hospitals will not succeed unless health care leaders committed to total quality motivate and lead medical staff beyond the "I don't have time" syndrome and help them realize the importance of this shift, preferably early on in the process. As the gatekeepers of the health care system — those who by law define, authorize, and carry out medical treatment — physicians must inevitably play a pivotal role in the future direction of health care

54

and the place of hospitals within the system as a whole. While I repeatedly stress to those in health care professions that total quality management is not primarily intended as a cost-cutting strategy but rather focuses on quality of care in terms of effectiveness, efficiency, and patient satisfaction, the influence of physicians on health care costs is very apparent and fundamental to succeeding with total quality management.

A strong advocate of total quality management as an important development in health care and supporter of physician involvement in continuous quality improvement projects, Dr. Paul Cooper, a St. Joseph's Health Centre neurologist and current vice-president of Medical Affairs, often refers to an observation by Dr. Robert McMurtry, the University of Western Ontario's dean of medicine, that approximately 70 per cent of the costs in hospitals directly and indirectly are the result of decisions made by doctors. "This, of course, is not an unusual figure, given that hospitals are the setting in which physicians, particularly specialists, conduct much of their practice," Dr. Cooper says. "But it is also a strong signal that in these days of deficits and shrinking resources, we must improve the efficiency and the effectiveness of the system if we are going to maintain high standards of medical care and prevent costs skyrocketing out of control. The wise and considered use of resources involves us as a profession."

PHYSICIANS' CURRENT SKEPTICISM

Physicians are skeptical these days, particularly when it comes to new ideas and strategies aimed at better management of what in their view is an increasingly conflictual health care environment. In recent years, many physicians have come to view management/physician relations, increased government scrutiny and control, and greater public demands for accountability as challenges to their professional autonomy and their ability to care for patients. Often physicians feel they are receiving the lion's share of the blame for the system's financial woes and service shortfalls; they are distressed by a troubling trend of doctor-bashing, where the inadequacies or wrongdoings of a few are held up as a reflection of the many.

A national survey of 3,387 Canadian physicians conducted by the Angus Reid Group for *The Medical Post* and released in the fall of 1992, indicates just how ingrained the "us versus them" mentality has become in health care, even between physicians and their own professional associations. More than half (59 per cent) of the survey respondents said they did not believe that their provincial medical associations gave good value for membership fees paid. And one-third of physicians nationwide said their provincial colleges were unsupportive. The biggest lumps, however, were delivered to governments — 81 per cent of physicians said provincial governments were unsupportive of the medical profession. Many also slammed the federal government — more than 70 per cent in every province ranked the federal government as not very supportive or not supportive at all.

So it should come as no surprise when hospital CEOs, convinced of the potential of total quality management to bring into being a positive future for hospitals, find that it is a hard sell to pessimistic physicians. "Many physicians have a deep distrust of clinical measurement projects initiated by management," writes Brent C. James of Intermountain Health Care Inc. in Utah, an organization regarded as a health care leader in total quality management. "That distrust has a well-established basis in experience. For several decades health care quality assurance programs have used inspection to identify — then punish — 'bad' practitioners. Some clinicians also perceive that most management-sponsored 'quality' projects are in fact thinly disguised efforts to reduce health care resource utilization, seemingly without regard for the potential impact of such actions on patients' health."[1]

I have yet to meet a physician who doesn't think that, at best, quality assurance has been a waste of their time. Needless to say, physicians do not perceive their work as a manufacturing process resulting in a product. Nor are they accustomed to thinking of patients as customers. And while physicians themselves expect a great number of services to be in place in hospitals to enable them to conduct their clinical practices, they are also not likely to see themselves in this context as both customer and supplier. Rather, suggests James, it is crucial to build support for total quality management in health care based upon established medical philosophy and practice that already embody many of the principles of continuous quality improvement. Physicians will generally not be receptive to total quality management if it is presented as a "new theory" borrowed from industry.

MAKING THE CASE FOR TQM

To put health care institutions on the path of total quality management, we have to convince physicians and other health care professionals who make up hospitals' diverse multidisciplinary treatment teams that total quality management is not simply another management flavour of the month. We also have to make a strong case to medical professionals that total quality management and the tools of continuous quality improvement can be relevant to clinical processes.

The best people to sell physicians on total quality management are other physicians, ones who have become convinced of its value and effectiveness. At St. Joseph's Health Centre and at other Canadian hospitals making progress with total quality management, such as the University of Alberta Hospitals in Edmonton, much attention was given to identifying physicians receptive to taking a leading role in creating change. It has been shown from a management perspective that total quality management must be led by senior management's visibility and commitment. So it is the case that in a hospital, in addition to management leadership, the commitment and cooperation of senior physicians in positions of leadership are needed. At St. Joseph's, among key senior medical staff who became involved early on were Dr. Paul Cooper; Dr. David Taylor, chief of emergency services; and Dr. Peter Cordy, a nephrologist and former chief of the Department of Medicine, vice-president of Medical Affairs, and who is now the Health Centre's first chairman of the Clinical Quality Task Force.

An integral part of the Health Centre's strategy was the development of a plan to introduce senior physicians to the concepts and tools of continuous quality improvement. Lectures and seminars were organized with speakers from both within and outside the Health Centre. Physicians received literature regarding continuous quality improvement, and since many physicians keep abreast of current developments in their field through reading journal articles written by their peers, both Cordy and Cooper undertook to produce articles on the relevance of continuous quality improvement to medical professionals.

In one of these articles, "Continuous Quality Improvement: The Role of the Medical Staff" published in the winter of 1992, Dr. Cordy succinctly summarized the urgency of why physicians need to get involved in the search for a better way in health care: "There is no question that the health care system in Canada is embarking upon a period of accelerated change, which will strain the capacity of all hospitals to respond. Health care funding will diminish in real terms, and there will be a growing emphasis on community care, ambulatory care, cost effectiveness, accountability and prevention. Acute-care beds will decrease by at least 20 per cent. In addition to these forces, teaching hospitals will have to adapt to the cutback in resources provided to the universities that results in reduced funding for medical staff engaged in teaching and research, the cost of which is often passed on to the hospitals. Furthermore, the reduction in resident staff will result in uncertainty and a change in roles, together with a need to replace residents with other healthcare providers. Although there have been substantial improvements in healthcare delivery in the past 10 years, the rate of external change in the future is likely to be such that most institutions will fail to thrive unless there is an organization-wide system to allow individuals and groups to respond."[2]

According to the 1992 Angus Reid/*Medical Post* survey of Canadian doctors, the majority of physicians anticipate increased external scrutiny of their standards and practices. In response to the question "Do you expect in 10 years funding bodies will scrutinize treatment patterns and require you to follow standard protocols?", 87 per cent replied yes. The survey also found that due to the rapid proliferation of medical and scientific knowledge, 64 per cent of physicians doubt they will be as on top of medical knowledge as they are today.

That the future holds dramatic changes in health care is not disputed by today's physicians, and if the Angus Reid/*Medical Post* survey is to be believed, they do not expect the changes to be positive. While 83 per cent of physicians rated Canada's current health care system as very good or excellent, two-thirds also felt that the Canadian system would significantly decline in the next 10 years unless changes were made, and 84 per cent believed that patient demand would outstrip the system's available financial resources.

What was interesting about this survey was that there were few suggestions offered for long-term improvements in the system, but instead a series of "quick fix" measures was proposed, such as a five-dollar user fee for patients visiting hospital emergency departments, an end to medicare coverage of plastic surgery categorized as "reconstructive," a "user pays" scheme for such reproductive technologies as in-vitro fertilization, and the "privatization" of hospitals. (*Medical Post* writers interpreted this to mean running hospitals "like microcorporations for greater efficiency." However, no one proposed how this could be done.) There was even some suggestion, by 40 per cent of survey respondents, that there should be some limits on coverage for illnesses and injuries that are "inflicted by persistently unhealthy habits," such as alcoholism.

I believe that much of this sense of loss of control over the direction of the system and its many complex problems could well be mitigated by physicians exploring the potential of the measurement and data-gathering tools of continuous quality improvement. These tools enable them to self-direct change and achieve data-driven results, rather than have such change imposed externally. The same data and measurement tools can also be effective in helping physicians to stay on top of their fields, because implicit in continuous quality improvement is the dynamic process of continuous learning, evaluation of what they do, and the search for a better way.

As well, organizational structures must change to enable hospital programs to be more responsive to the environment and the demands to alter the ways we care for the patient. It will take a bold group of leaders to reshape our slow, awkward and frustrating organizations. We know that small groups are more responsive to a reshaping process that will result in greater degrees of freedom for programs while ensuring that these programs remain focused on the vision and goals created for them.

INVOLVING PHYSICIANS FROM THE OUTSET

In his book *Curing Health Care*, Donald Berwick, himself a physician, observes that the involvement of physicians in total quality management is one of the formidable challenges a hospital has to meet. "Institutions launching quality improvement programs almost always ask: How shall we involve doctors, who do not seem to see themselves as players in processes, whose financial incentives impede participation in project teams and data collection activities, and who do not strongly believe that their interests are tied to the improvement of the health care organizations they work in? In fact, barriers to physician involvement may turn out to be the most important single issue impeding the success of quality improvement in medical care."[3]

According to Berwick, the key is to convince physicians that many of their own interests are served by participating in continuous quality improvement initiatives. "They must understand that better processes mean for them less frustration, less risk, and higher productive capacity," Berwick writes. "They must actually experience the benefits of improved customer-supplier relationships. And they must be helped to understand, if at all possible, why their own futures are connected to the health of the organizations in which care is given. It is the job of leaders — clinical and nonclinical — to explain this."4

Many of the U.S. health care organizations that have started total quality management initially perhaps took an inappropriate turn, which is making their journey longer. They began with nonclinical continuous quality improvement projects because they believed it would be difficult to involve physicians until it could be proven that CQI works. As Brent James describes the situation, early attempts to apply total quality management within health care tended to focus on problems with hospital support services or medical infrastructure. In that context, physicians did not perceive their own important role in assuring that patients have a positive experience at the receiving end of hospital support services; indeed, they were deeply suspicious of the whole process.

"Some groups, drawing upon the teachings of industrial quality control, tried to generate detailed specifications for health care process steps," observes James. "They usually used care protocols developed by external consensus panels or through small internal groups. But independent physicians fear the loss of clinical control that such standardized protocols imply. They also distrust management's motives in introducing new control mechanisms. Therefore, the resulting protocols were often ignored."5

Stumbling blocks such as James describes underscore the importance of involving physicians in total quality management *at the outset*. Hospitals that cannot elicit the co-operation and involvement of physicians in total quality management risk having their physicians develop hostility to changes in which they are not involved and which they do not fully understand.

I recall one physician who was involved in one of the first clinical continuous quality improvement process teams. He was often considered a skeptic or a cynic, given his history with administration where the program-of-the-year approach frequently frustrated him and other physicians because of lack of results. But he reluctantly became part of the team. Six months later, I bumped into him at the squash club. He began talking about the team's results, which were fairly successful, and suggested that "every physician needs to go through this process, because there's so much to learn and to improve upon in medical practice." He and others who were part of the early clinical continuous quality improvement project teams are now our greatest advocates.

Among the key areas identified at St. Joseph's Health Centre in which total quality management would have an impact upon physicians and clinical teams were maintaining levels of service, shifting inpatient surgery to outpatient, expanding ambulatory care, and shortening average length of stay. Viewed as crucial aspects of organizational revitalization, they needed to be fully linked to both the hospital's strategic plan and its fiscal strategy. In outpatient surgery, for example, currently about 70 per cent of surgical procedures at St. Joseph's Health Centre are performed on an outpatient basis. If, as I observed in Chapter Two, we are at the end of the hospitalization era, part of the new vision for health care means achieving even higher outpatient surgery rates which accomplish both satisfactory results for patients and are cost effective. The "tools of quality" needed for the future were defined at St. Joseph's as the development of systematic critical analysis of all processes of care. In 1990, when I presented the notion to a group of ambulatory-care managers that 70 per cent of surgery could be performed on an outpatient basis by 1995, I was met with disbelief. It is now 1993 and the 70 per cent has already been achieved — 80 per cent is probably only three to five years away.

Rather than become discouraged by the initial skepticism of physicians and other medical staff, hospitals can view this skepticism as a potential strength to help make the shift toward total quality management. Almost every physician, nurse, or any other health professional, can tell you about his or her frustrations with the current system within an individual hospital and in the system as a whole, and most will say there is an urgent need for a better way.

"I have all these patients waiting for their operations," says one surgeon. "They are all sick, they need the surgery, and many have to be on waiting lists. Maybe their condition worsens during this time. Certainly their quality of life is no great shakes while they're waiting. It's an awful thing to be left hanging like that. As for my position, I feel caught between the constraints in the system and the needs of my patients — and this is stressful for all concerned. The surgical team, the nurses, we all feel pressured by the huge demand on us to care for the full house of patients we have, and we feel equally pressured by the knowledge of all those who are waiting and whom we just can't get to as quickly as we would like."

As organizational research and analysis shows, often expressed as Deming's 85/15 rule, most (85 per cent of) obstacles to good service and productivity lie in process problems, not in people. In other words, long patient waiting lists may have more to do with system inefficiencies than with the "slowness" of people to get things done or, for that matter, governments who "underfund" the system. Indeed, many of the reasons for slowness will be found in unnecessary or redundant steps in the work processes.

When doctors and patients alike express frustration at the lack of available beds, the solutions may lie in more effective discharge planning or on strategies aimed at achieving shorter lengths of stay that are just as safe for patients as the longer current ones. In the words of organizational consultant and professor of organizational behaviour and management at Boston University, George Labovitz, whose work involves helping many health care organizations design quality strategies, "You can't get them in if you can't get them out."

In industry, system inefficiencies and waste can account for 20 to 30 per cent of gross sales. Several hospital CEOs have also noted similar inefficiencies in health care — that 25 to 30 per cent of what is done in hospitals does not add value to patient processes. In other words, it is waste. At a round-table discussion at the Toronto "Owning the Future: The Landmark Forum on CQI" conference in October 1992, sponsored jointly by St. Joseph's Health Centre and the University of Toronto Department of Health Administration, William MacLeod, CEO of Women's College Hospital in Toronto, described total quality management as "a method to recapture that waste."

St. Joseph's Dr. Paul Cooper believes physicians must be convinced of the value of CQI not just in making hospitals as a whole run more efficiently, but also their own individual practices, since it takes time both to learn the concepts and tools of CQI and to participate in CQI projects, and for most physicians time is money. "One of the selling points I use when talking with other physicians about this," says Dr. Cooper, "is to suggest that they see this time/money as an investment in a better future. It will pay itself back in the increased efficiency and effectiveness of our treatment programs. It allows us to keep doing what we do best for our patients, and it becomes easier to deliver service better."

The result is win-win. Rather than being the victims of external constraints, clinical teams can take hold of the process, measure what works and what does not, identify barriers to quality and service, and implement change that is backed up by solid data and stands up to scrutiny, internal or external.

SCIENTIFIC METHODOLOGY IS AT THE HEART OF CQI

Total quality management can be embedded effectively into medical practice if there is a will to do so, because when you get past the initial strangeness of the language, you uncover a congruence of values. George Labovitz observes that total quality management may be more natural to health care than even to industry or business because the practices of the majority of health care professionals are value-based in concepts of service, care, and compassion for the sick and injured.

Medical staff in general already have a genuine commitment to quality. "The medical profession requires that its members routinely evaluate and improve the quality of the medical care they deliver," writes Brent James. "In traditional medical practice, quality assurance takes place through 'peer review' — a group of clinical peers with fundamental knowledge regarding the disease and treatment in question reviews a physician's performance, looking for mistakes or opportunities for improvement."[6]

Another natural extension of medical practice into total quality management is that physicians and other medical professionals within current health care practice have become accustomed to working in multidisciplinary teams. The complexity of health care and the rapid pace of new health care knowledge practically ensure that the days of the independent sole practitioner in hospitals are fading. The care of patients in hospitals now routinely involves not only referrals and consultations among medical specialties, but the skills and input of many other health professionals, such as clinical nurse specialists or physiotherapists, as well as the skills and talents of support staff.

The field of biomedical research has also undergone significant change in the direction of cross-functional research teams. Gone is the solitary scientist closeted in a laboratory. "Collaborations among basic scientists such as physiologists or physicists and clinical scientists — doctors who conduct research — have become increasingly the norm," says Dr. John Challis, the director of St. Joseph's Health Centre's research facility, the Lawson Research Institute. "Research institutes, whether free-standing or attached to hospitals, are now designed to enable interdisciplinary research. International collaborations among research centres are also becoming far more frequent."

At the "Owning the Future" conference, George Labovitz observed during one of the sessions that medical research, with its mandate to "find a better way" and its collaborative efforts among areas as diverse as magnetic resonance imaging and molecular biology, is a model of continuous quality improvement in action. Comments Labovitz, "We need to learn from *them*."

The methods of continuous quality improvement appeal also to physicians' commitment to the use of the scientific method and the gathering of reliable data. At the centre of continuous quality improvement is the use of data collection and measurement that yield concrete findings. The process of CQI is compatible with scientific methods in the practice of medicine, and can be framed within the context of scientific discipline:

1. Observe the process.
2. Identify the steps in the process.
3. Measure current performance.
4. Make hypotheses for improvement.
5. Put changes into effect.
6. Test the results of change.

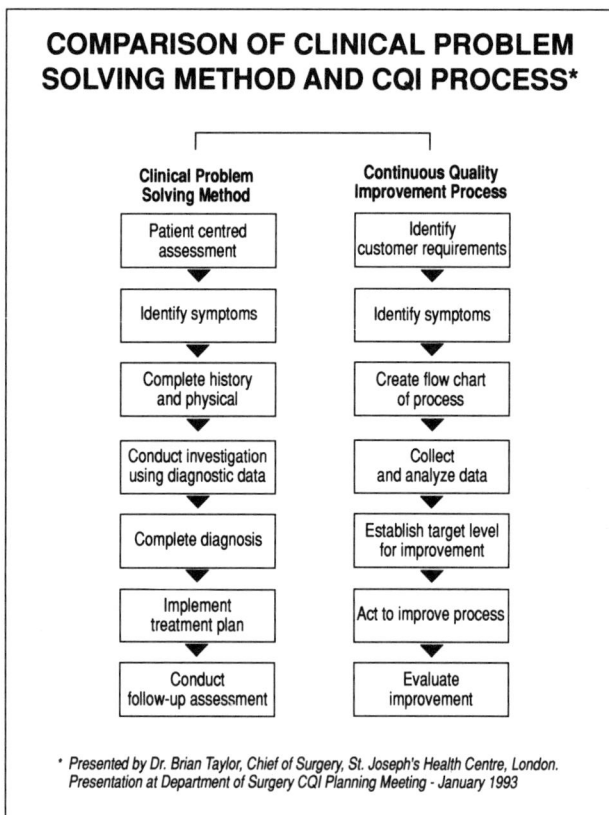

COMPARISON OF CLINICAL PROBLEM SOLVING METHOD AND CQI PROCESS*

Clinical Problem Solving Method	Continuous Quality Improvement Process
Patient centred assessment	Identify customer requirements
Identify symptoms	Identify symptoms
Complete history and physical	Create flow chart of process
Conduct investigation using diagnostic data	Collect and analyze data
Complete diagnosis	Establish target level for improvement
Implement treatment plan	Act to improve process
Conduct follow-up assessment	Evaluate improvement

Presented by Dr. Brian Taylor, Chief of Surgery, St. Joseph's Health Centre, London. Presentation at Department of Surgery CQI Planning Meeting - January 1993

"There is room for optimism, since we know from the work of NDP [National Demonstration Project] teams and others that, once involved in teams, physicians enjoy the quality improvement process as much as any participants," writes Donald Berwick. "The scientific methods at the heart of process improvement are familiar to them. The same methods are the foundation for sound clinical research and evaluation, and, to some extent, they are the methods of good clinical practice itself. In the day-to-day work of the doctor, ideally, patients come with needs, physicians and others collect and interpret data on the pathophysiologic processes, physicians formulate treatment plans, and patients and physicians together monitor and adjust their subsequent activities based on the feedback. This sequence, relabelled, is the general problem-solving sequence followed by any well-trained quality improvement project team. In short, the challenge of involving physicians in quality improvement may lie primarily at the beginning of the effort; once involved, physicians can be quality champions of the first order."[7]

If the tools and strategies of continuous quality improvement, and the larger philosophy of total quality management, can be successfully linked to physicians' needs, not only in their treatment processes but in the organizational processes required to carry out patient care, medical staff and senior management can then work together to achieve positive and lasting change. This begins to address the question "What's in it for physicians?" Much of the "us versus them" conflict then becomes a dinosaur.

Dr. Bernard Badley, CEO of Victoria General Hospital in Halifax, feels that his experience as a physician and then as an administrator embodies both the past "us versus them" and the future possibility of collaborative solutions to many health care system problems. When he was a practising physician, one of his "hobbies," he says, was habitually criticizing hospital management for the bureaucratic obstacles getting in the way of medical practice. When he transferred to an administrative role, the traditional management methods dominant at the time were those of exhortation, control, and organizational hierarchy. But in CQI, as it is being implemented at Victoria General, he sees the antithesis of that model and in its place "a new vision and tools . . . to unlock the potential of smart people in hospitals."

In order to evaluate clinical processes, we need measurement tools adapted to health care environments. As a key starting point, the evaluative tool value improvement program (VIP) has proved highly useful at St. Joseph's and several other hospitals, such as Foothills in Calgary and the University of Alberta Hospitals. Later, as VIP projects began to trigger ideas for other clinical improvement initiatives, St. Joseph's began framing improvement projects involving patient-care programs as clinical continuous quality improvement (CCQI).

HOW WELL ARE WE DOING CLINICALLY?

In Chapter Two I discussed briefly the VIP projects undertaken at Foothills Provincial General Hospital during my time there. Projects focusing on total hip replacement, myocardial infarction, cataract surgery, and gallbladder surgery were successful in achieving significant reductions in length of stay, positive patient outcomes, and good cost savings. Prior to the official launch of total quality management at St. Joseph's Health Centre, CCQI projects played a crucial role in the development of methods for measuring clinical quality.

VIP is a resource management tool to review possible changes in care giver practices and behaviours without negatively affecting the quality of care. By defining quality of care as the capacity to offer the patient the greatest achievable health benefits with minimum unnecessary risks and the use of resources in ways satisfactory to the patient, we can identify four determinants of quality care: outcome, safety, cost, and patient satisfaction.

VIP was developed initially by Baxter Corporation (U.S.) as a process in part to improve customer/supplier relations. In health care, it has evolved into an evaluative tool that uses a multidisciplinary approach to deal with the analysis of issues that have the potential to bring about cost savings without adversely affecting quality of care. In many instances, quality is actually enhanced as a result of this process. From a total quality management perspective, I feel it is important to emphasize that although VIP is structured to identify potential cost savings, its value for continuous quality improvement is much greater, for it allows every aspect of care — from admission to discharge — to be evaluated in great detail. Many opportunities for improvements in service and patient satisfaction are uncovered through VIP.

A value improvement program can, in fact, be a very constructive tool in linking the necessity of cost effectiveness with commitment to quality of care. Now more than at any other time, hospitals have a greater need to work together with all levels of the organization to ensure that the resources entrusted to them are focused primarily on the needs of patients.

Macro-level reviews of resource utilization have been only marginally successful in addressing rising health care costs. The traditional method of balancing hospital budgets — closing beds — has not had the effect of reducing health care costs in the long run. It has, however, served to work against the best interests of patients and their physicians.

Hospitals need a microscopic multidisciplinary tool that leads to savings and promotes quality. VIP, as an analytical process, shows promising results, particularly in terms of involving medical staff. Significant gains are possible for hospitals through the successful use of VIP techniques. Both the Alberta and Ontario government funding systems, for example, allow hospitals to take advantage of built-in incentives for increased efficiency and productivity. Since a major portion of costs are accounted for in the room and care category, efforts to decrease length of stay have been instrumental in realizing savings opportunities.

When hospitals select a clinical procedure to study, the following factors are important to the choice of project:

1. the level of interest and commitment of the physician leader
2. annual treatment volume
3. level of comparability across hospitals
4. transferability of recommendations to other areas (halo or ripple effect)
5. availability of a data base for comparison.

In early 1991, St. Joseph's began two studies: uncomplicated cholecystectomy (gallbladder removal), and normal labour and delivery. There are various models of VIP, but all generally follow the same process and include a detailed costing model. The first task is to develop a patient profile for the study area. In the case of the cholecystectomy study, this was gallbladder patients under 55 with no complications, such as diabetes. Then followed a chart review of 20 to 25 patients who fit these criteria. The review looked at areas such as length of stay, tests performed, room and care, surgery, supplies, drugs, and IVs.

Each of those areas was assessed in terms of cost. The data were then compared with similar assessments of the same procedure in other hospitals, and using the most cost-effective practice in each category, an "ideal procedure" was created. The process allowed St. Joseph's to measure how well it did in terms of costs compared to similar hospitals, and to analyse the causes of deviation from the ideal composite.

St. Joseph's overall cost for gallbladder surgery was, at $1,774 a patient, lower than that of all the comparison Canadian and U.S. hospitals. Labour and delivery, at $1,397, was also found to be lower. The purpose of these processes is not, however, always to adopt the least expensive practice in a certain category. If, in the judgment of the clinical team, patients are better served by more resources being spent in a certain category, then that is what the team adopts as its practice. For example, if sending patients home two days earlier than was previously the norm resulted in significant numbers of these patients having to be readmitted to hospital because of complications, the clinical team would adopt the length of stay that appears to assure the best health outcome for the patient *the first time,* which is one of the key principles of total quality management. It is vital that the teams have freedom to choose the best way to deliver quality care *based on data.* Every place I have used this model, the teams have always chosen such that costs are *never* greater and quality is *always* higher.

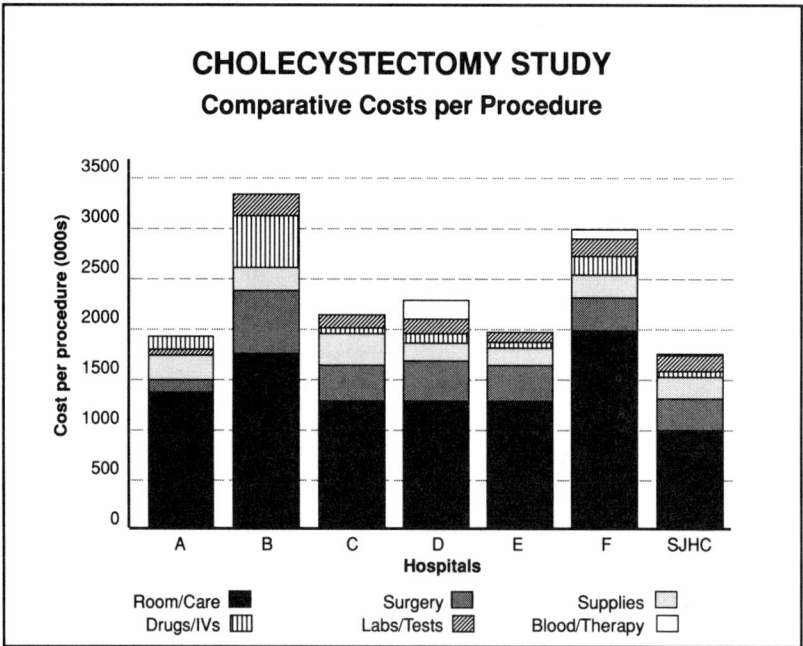

CHOLECYSTECTOMY STUDY
Comparative Costs per Procedure

Significant opportunities for both improvement and cost reduction were identified by the teams. For example, eliminating routine chest X-rays on admission except for patients for whom the procedure is deemed necessary (that is, if the patient has a history of respiratory problems or on admission appears to have a respiratory infection) resulted in savings of $3,600 in the cholecystectomy program, and through the ripple effect to other surgical procedures was capable of realizing savings of $21,000. A change in the way antibiotics were prescribed before surgery resulted in a saving of $1,900 to the cholecystectomy program and global saving of $41,000.

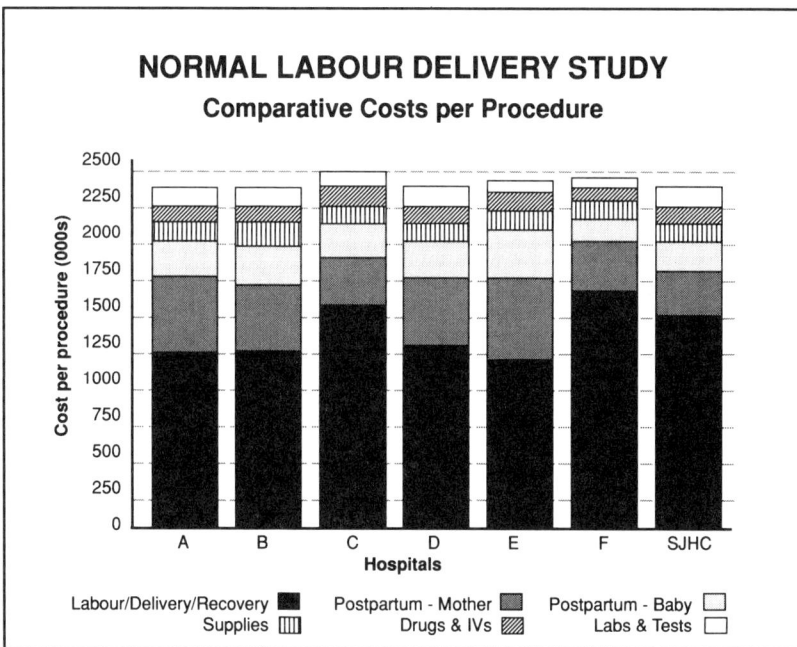

NORMAL LABOUR DELIVERY STUDY
Comparative Costs per Procedure

Cost per procedure (000s)

Hospitals: A B C D E F SJHC

Labour/Delivery/Recovery ■   Postpartum - Mother ▨   Postpartum - Baby ☐
Supplies ▥   Drugs & IVs ▨   Labs & Tests ☐

Routine laboratory urinalysis was replaced by a "dipstick" test, with only "suspicious" results going on for further investigation. This resulted in a saving of about $1,500 to cholecystectomy and a global saving of $45,000, shared with the labour and delivery study. The elimination of routine complete blood-count post-operative testing, except for certain specific patients, accomplished a saving of approximately $4,000 to cholecystectomy and a global saving of $25,000.

It was also noted by the medical and nursing staff that it is not necessary to replace post-operative dressings following their removal after it was determined that patients who do not have their dressings replaced are no more at risk of infection than patients who do. This change in the use of supplies brought $12,000 in savings to the cholecystectomy study and $49,000 in global savings when transferred to other surgical procedures.

These were only a few of the process improvements accomplished by the clinical continuous quality improvement efforts. Not only were potential cost savings realized, but more importantly, the changes had positive effects on the organization as a whole and on patient outcomes and satisfaction. For example, lower numbers of routine urinalysis and complete blood-count tests have helped eliminate unnecessary testing and allowed for a more manageable — and therefore more efficient — workload in the labs. From the patient's point of view, it has meant not being stuck one too many times with a needle or, in the case of reduced numbers of chest X-rays, less unnecessary exposure to radiation. Changes in antibiotic prescription procedures served both to reduce patient drug intake and to ensure effective protection from post-operative infections.

In every case, the doctors and other care givers were very pleased with the quality improvements made. While some of the procedures involved in gallbladder surgery have been superseded by the newer laparoscopic cholecystectomy method (belly-button surgery), many of the recommendations (for example, concerning lab tests and the use of antibiotics) still apply, and to numerous other surgical procedures, as well.

The recommendations from the task force for cholecystectomy also spurred the expansion of St. Joseph's preadmission same-day surgery program for patients admitted for elective surgery. Jean, a 42-year-old mother of two, described her relief at being able to spend the night before her surgery in the comfort of her home. Previously she would have had to spend a stressful first day in hospital undergoing tests and preparations for surgery. Now these preparations are accomplished on an outpatient basis, and Jean can be admitted straight to the floor on the day of her surgery rather than having to go through admitting. The preadmission program has resulted in increasing patient satisfaction and decreasing average length of stay, while reducing room and care costs.

Physician involvement in such clinical evaluation projects is imperative. Among clinical professionals, a physician's relationship with hospital administration is unique under the current way health care is funded in Canada. The majority of physicians are not directly employed by the hospital, yet they exercise enormous control over the hospital's resources. When doctors are involved with meetings and other team activities, such as clinical evaluation projects, they cannot bill for the time. This negative financial impact can be a major source of resistance.

Although their involvement is limited by an adverse impact on their time and incomes, most physicians have demonstrated that their financial goals are secondary to the assurance of high-quality medical outcomes for their patients. When project team members show sensitivity to this time/financial impact upon physicians and schedule meetings to best meet everyone's needs, physicians come on board quickly. A similar sensitivity must be accorded to other medical professionals on the project team as well, such as nurses and therapists, who, while they are salaried and do not have the same loss-of-income concerns, are nevertheless pressured for time in the face of enormous patient-care demands. These team members also do not get extra staff coverage while away at team meetings.

Success with CCQI has spurred a number of other clinically based projects at St. Joseph's, most recently a CCQI project for dialysis and one for cataract surgery. CCQI is only one of a number of analysis approaches that can be used to achieve improvements in clinical quality.

St. Joseph's medical staff has also played a key role in three of the hospital's initial continuous quality improvement demonstration projects dealing with three "high pain" patient-care areas: a radiology team to improve the efficiency and reliability of the film library in order to prevent delays from loss of X-ray films, often resulting in X-rays being reordered; a project to reduce patient waiting time in the emergency department through innovations such as "fast tracking"; and an operating room/surgical day care unit/post-anaesthetic care unit team working on reducing the length of patients' waits, from the time they are called from the patient rooms to the operating room. (This last project has an excess of 100 steps done 80 times a day and, in almost all hospitals, is problematic.)

Other clinical improvement teams are studying the use of episiotomies — a "routine" incision performed on a woman's perineal area to assist her in giving birth — with a view to reducing the number of inappropriate episiotomies; medical/surgical discharge planning to shorten gaps between actual and expected time of patient discharge; and complex-cases discharge planning to ensure timely, safe, and efficient discharge of patients requiring complex care.

The Western Ontario Provincial Lithotripsy Program, located at St.

Joseph's, was designed from the outset with a customer focus. The clinical service and communications strategies have been refined in response to customer needs. The number of preliminary tests patients must undergo has been reduced, the physician referral network has been streamlined, and patients now receive additional information to help them feel comfortable with the procedure. There is more about our demonstration projects, and newer project teams in Chapter Five.

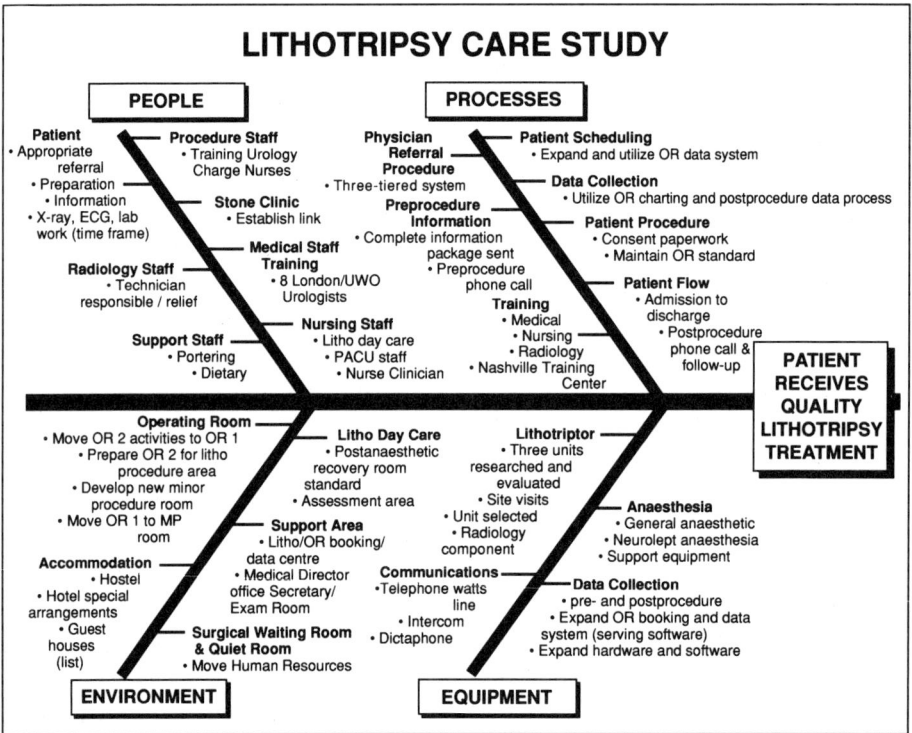

LITHOTRIPSY CARE STUDY

PEOPLE

PROCESSES

Patient
- Appropriate referral
- Preparation
- Information
- X-ray, ECG, lab work (time frame)

Procedure Staff
- Training Urology Charge Nurses

Stone Clinic
- Establish link

Radiology Staff
- Technician responsible / relief

Medical Staff Training
- 8 London/UWO Urologists

Support Staff
- Portering
- Dietary

Nursing Staff
- Litho day care
- PACU staff
- Nurse Clinician

Physician Referral Procedure
- Three-tiered system

Preprocedure Information
- Complete information package sent
- Preprocedure phone call

Training
- Medical
- Nursing
- Radiology
- Nashville Training Center

Patient Scheduling
- Expand and utilize OR data system

Data Collection
- Utilize OR charting and postprocedure data process

Patient Procedure
- Consent paperwork
- Maintain OR standard

Patient Flow
- Admission to discharge
- Postprocedure phone call & follow-up

PATIENT RECEIVES QUALITY LITHOTRIPSY TREATMENT

Operating Room
- Move OR 2 activities to OR 1
- Prepare OR 2 for litho procedure area
- Develop new minor procedure room
- Move OR 1 to MP room

Accommodation
- Hostel
- Hotel special arrangements
- Guest houses (list)

Litho Day Care
- Postanaesthetic recovery room standard
- Assessment area

Support Area
- Litho/OR booking/data centre
- Medical Director office Secretary/Exam Room

Surgical Waiting Room & Quiet Room
- Move Human Resources

Lithotriptor
- Three units researched and evaluated
- Site visits
- Unit selected
- Radiology component

Communications
- Telephone watts line
- Intercom
- Dictaphone

Anaesthesia
- General anaesthetic
- Neurolept anaesthesia
- Support equipment

Data Collection
- pre- and postprocedure
- Expand OR booking and data system (serving software)
- Expand hardware and software

ENVIRONMENT

EQUIPMENT

Both the lithotripsy program and the emergency department's clinical improvement project were highlighted at the October 1992 "Owning the Future" conference. Representatives from a number of Canadian hospitals shared some of their experiences and results with quality improvement projects aimed at patient care. At the University of Alberta Hospitals (UAH), for example, to date there have been more than 100 project teams. Some early successes include a 21.2 per cent reduction in resources required to perform total hip replacement and a 23.1 per cent reduction in resources required to perform gallbladder surgery. Recently, they have developed a new way of drawing blood from children who have central lines implanted to allow for treatments such as chemotherapy; it involves the innovation of applying in the line a Y-connector port, which makes the procedure less painful and less risky. Besides also being almost 50 per cent less costly, this new blood-collection process allows the procedure to be done while the child is asleep. The child does not have to be held down forcibly, nor does the whole IV line need to be opened, which greatly lessens the chance of infection.

University of Alberta Hospitals has also adopted, on a wide scale, a system of clinical review called "objective occurrence screening" aimed at measuring both the quality and appropriateness of care. Patient records are screened within 48 hours of the patient's admission, then every 48 to 72 hours during hospital stay, and finally at post-discharge. Using objective criteria, experienced nurses trained as clinical-care analysts identify from the records any adverse occurrences related to patient care, process, and outcomes.

Not only does the process uncover out-of-the-ordinary occurrences or other situations that should be addressed, it also begins to identify differences in patterns of practice so that these patterns can then be analysed in terms of appropriateness and effectiveness. UAH has introduced this program to approximately nine of its departments, including pediatrics, nephrology, general surgery, and cardiology.

Some of the things watched for in objective occurrences screening are a patient requiring admission to hospital as a result of an outpatient procedure, drug use that is inappropriate or excessive, a hospital-acquired infection, and excessive blood loss. For example, a child being treated for a sinus infection was also found to be anemic, but no action was taken or further blood work done to discover the cause. Another situation was that blood tests to measure electrolytes were frequently being performed on the same patients several times. Dr. Ronald Wensel, who presented UAH's objective occurrence screening program at the conference, said that often the reason for many adverse occurrences can be traced to system problems. In the case of the electrolyte tests, for example, it was the lab's slow turnaround time (a common problem in many hospitals) in getting results back to the floor, a situation that then caused the physician to reorder the test and its results stat, that is, right away.

The fact that this outcome evaluation is being conducted concurrently with the patient's admission to hospital has resulted in the process picking up 85 per cent of adverse or questionable outcomes, Dr. Wensel informed the conference attendees, as opposed to 15 per cent when the evaluation is done retrospectively — that is, after the patient has left the hospital or been transferred somewhere else.

St. Joseph's Health Centre physicians are also looking at implementing similar concurrent clinical evaluations and are exploring how this can best be done. It could be that evaluating every chart, as is done at UAH, is too costly in terms of trained staff to conduct the evaluations and the time it takes to do them. If departments were instead to evaluate samplings of patients and focus primarily on the four or so most common procedures for that department, the 85 per cent success rate at picking up adverse outcomes may well be achieved.

MEDICAL STAFF INVOLVEMENT MUST BE PLANNED AND ONGOING

St. Joseph's Health Centre physicians are now at the stage of what some of their colleagues have identified as "informed pessimism." There is a certain amount of resistance and skepticism, but also a real desire to change direction and an increasing openness to participate on quality improvement teams. Pressures on physicians' time from the university, the Health Centre committee responsibilities, and most importantly, the sheer volume of patient load, often make it difficult for physicians to focus on a long-term vision for the Health Centre that embodies significant transformational change.

In his book *Creating Culture Change: The Key to Successful Total Quality Management*, Philip Atkinson describes two different orientations in organizations: Transactors and Transformers. Transactors are people- and task-centred; they emphasize the practical and concrete, maintain stability in the environment, and seek tangible results. Transformers are forward-planning, visionary and inspirational, creative, open to challenge, and oriented to change.

"Frankly, I see myself much more in the Transactor role," writes Dr. Paul Cooper in a planning document for the involvement of St. Joseph's physicians in continuous quality improvement, "and I believe that the vast majority of physicians in the Health Centre would fall into that category.

"I see Phil [Hassen] much more in the Transformer role, and I think that one of our tasks is to get some of the Transformational 'Vision' inspiring the Transactional role of ourselves and of the physicians."

In the spring of 1992, St. Joseph's held a two-part strategic-planning meeting with representatives from across the hospital, reflecting the cross-functional emphasis of total quality management. This included department chiefs, division heads, program directors, medical staff executive, managers, directors, board members, union representatives, and vice-presidents. This approach, which is becoming more and more the norm at St. Joseph's, supports the continued dialogue among clinical staff, administration, and other key stakeholders.

"The addition of MDs, etc. is the greatest!" wrote one of the participants in an evaluation of the meeting. "The old barriers seem to have disappeared — admin., medical staff, nursing staff, and others are truly collaborating," wrote another. And still another commented, "Very good to see physician participation throughout the day. Some are truly collaborative and interdisciplinary but *many* are trying very hard to involve others in their planning/practice. Very satisfying."

This is not to say, however, that at that meeting we had all arrived at a commitment to total quality management. Participants also identified the need for clearer directional statements and pointed out the lack of knowledge many departments have of each other. Others were worried about burnout, and still others wondered about whether the complexity of the organization would make it virtually impossible to have clinical and nonclinical staff truly share a vision of total quality management. Perhaps you can begin to understand why this transformation will take us and every other hospital many years to achieve the profound results total quality management can produce.

Also in the spring of 1992, Dr. Martin Merry, a physician from the University of New Hampshire, a 3M affiliate consultant, and a leader in quality improvement development, met with physicians and administrative leaders at St. Joseph's. Dr. Merry found that among the physicians who attended "there was good basic understanding of continuous improvement principles." He also identified, however, the natural inclination for physicians to want "more outside examples" from other institutions. He recommended that physicians focus instead on "home grown" projects rather than copying other institutions. One of the greatest strengths in strategies of continuous quality improvement are the tools that allow teams to focus on *their particular health care delivery situation.*

Continuous quality improvement works because improvement opportunities arise organically out of the process being analysed.

Dr. Merry's written summary of the meeting identified the state of informed pessimism that characterizes many St. Joseph's physicians and likely a good number of physicians in other hospitals making the shift to total quality management and continuous quality improvement:

> Another factor may be inhibiting presently knowledgeable physicians from taking a more vocal or visible teaching role in CQI development. CQI is a management, not clinical, process. During early stages of development, the majority of physicians on any medical staff will be skeptical of CQI. This is especially true if, as is almost always the case, the decision to develop CQI originates with administration. Physicians may participate individually on CQI projects and come to understand and accept the value of CQI techniques. They may even be willing to discuss their support for such projects in relatively private settings. But to become a visible change agent is likely to pose a risk to one's esteem among colleagues . . . As long as some physicians continue to express negativism toward CQI (such commonly heard 'charges' as 'administrative plot, passing fad,' etc.) a supportive physician risks approbation (possibly silent but nonetheless real) among his colleagues for his support. This phenomenon is normal, a form of generic resistance which accompanies any major change. Nonetheless, specific strategies to overcome it may be necessary.[8]

In other words, physicians are no different from other members of any organization undergoing significant change. Anxiety, fear, and confusion are part of the "crazy time" that must be slowly transformed to feelings of challenge, energy, and commitment. Simply put, given the pivotal role physicians occupy in hospitals, a strategy to involve them positively in CQI must be designed specifically for them.

Noting that at St. Joseph's several physicians were visibly enthusiastic about their CQI efforts, Dr. Merry suggested they become role models and internal teachers. He also recommended that hospital leaders continue their willingness to publicize and visibly communicate support for quality improvement throughout the Health Centre.

In the fall of 1992, Health Centre senior physicians with a basic understanding of continuous quality improvement concepts developed a number of presentations on clinical continuous quality improvement designed especially for, but not limited to, physicians. In addition, all physicians new to the Health Centre receive an introduction to quality improvement concepts. The progress of quality improvement projects are reported to the Medical Advisory Committee and there are articles frequently circulated about CQI. These are methods to communicate information to medical staff quickly and concisely, and not cut into their clinical time with patients or into their various research activities.

A further challenge is to expand the role of the old Audit Committee to include quality indicators in its mandate as a way of spurring wider interest in CQI activity. St. Joseph's has, as a result, formed a Clinical Quality Committee chaired by Dr. Peter Cordy, a senior physician. The committee will identify opportunities for clinical quality improvement projects throughout the hospital and will encourage the active involvement of physicians in leadership roles on these and other departmentally initiated projects.

Since one of the major complaints clinical staff have about committing to the vision of total quality management in health care is the time involved with projects (particularly time spent in meetings), the number of committees of the Medical Advisory Committee have been reduced from 22 to nine. For nursing, 12 committees have been reduced to five.

If I have any encouraging advice for other hospitals contemplating how best to gain the support of medical staff for total quality management as it applies to clinical areas, it is to be patient, persistent, and willing to live with a certain degree of flack while bridges of communication are built between administration and medical staff and while quality improvement teams gain experience in functioning across departments and focusing on all factors that affect a patient from admission to discharge.

We need to use a light hand in this type of change — leading, but not pushing. When we did the labour and delivery project, the physicians did not at that time adopt one of the important suggested changes — to stop routine cord gases. There were significant potential savings involved, but for clinical reasons the physicians were strongly opposed. However, of eleven key practices components, ten did change. Had we pushed for the eleventh, it would have had the potential effect of "inoculating" the physicians against CCQI for possibly years to come.

CLINICAL QUALITY IMPROVEMENT IS LINKED
TO WIDER HEALTH CARE ISSUES

At the level of individual hospitals, when clinical staff begin working with the tools of continuous quality improvement in addition to the medical-audit and peer-review processes that are already in place, often aspects of procedures are identified as either unnecessary or inappropriate. The decision not to replace post-operative surgical dressings as a result of the findings of St. Joseph's gallbladder surgery team is an example of how change was implemented when the medical team realized it made good sense to do so.

However, there are a great number of variations and practice prefer-ences among physicians across Canada, across North America, between other countries, and even within the same city, observes Dr. Cooper. One physician may prefer to keep patients in hospital two days longer than another. One prefers surgery as a first-line treatment for a certain condi-tion; another first tries medications or diet/exercise changes.

On the macro-level, differences in practice patterns among geograph-ical areas and countries have been identified for decades. You are much more likely to have your gallbladder out in Canada than in Great Britain. Rates of caesarian section are lower in many European countries than they are in North America. You are more likely to have your prostate surgically removed in Saskatchewan than in Alberta.[9]

The RAND Corporation in the U.S. has estimated that about 45 per cent of heart bypass surgery operations may be of dubious benefit to either quality or longevity of life. The patient group for whom heart bypass surgery is likely most appropriate are those requiring triple bypass, such as Allan Tyson whom you read about in Chapter One. But many patients who do not have the same degree of artery blockage that Allan Tyson had are also given bypass surgery when in fact more conservative methods of managing their conditions could well have been the best course of action. If there were more consensus concerning the appropriateness of this surgical procedure, Allan Tyson and other patients for whom this proce-dure *is* necessary may not have to encounter such long waiting lists. Interestingly, the U.S. does twice as many bypass operations per 100,000 people in its "no wait" system.

The issue of practice pattern variation and arguments/evidence for the appropriateness of certain procedures as opposed to others is enormously complex, having to take into account factors such as demography, morbidity, randomness, the availability of resources or supply, clinical judgment of medical professionals, patient expectation or demand, prevailing custom, rates for previous years of organ removal, omissions from data sources, and inaccuracies in data sources.[10] As such, in the interests of the length and focus of this book, a detailed discussion of these issues will not be raised here.

However, one key point to consider is that as macro-strategies at cost containment have proven ineffective in health care, continuous quality improvement strategies within health institutions appear to hold more promise in actually getting results. So, too, it may be the case that clinical continuous quality initiatives within health institutions may yield more data-supported consensus concerning medical practice variation than attempts at broader analysis have achieved to date.

The editor of the *New England Journal of Medicine*, Arnold Relman, has depicted the 1990s as an era of assessment and accountability in health care. Medical peer-review and quality-assurance models have long existed in hospitals, but since both these strategies tend to be retrospective in nature — that is, they look back at what has happened rather than analysing what *is* happening — their usefulness is thought by many to be limited in dealing with the complexities of modern health care.

In *Quality of Care: Issues and Challenges in the 90s*, recently published by the Canadian Medical Association, author MaryLou Harrigan identifies total quality management with its strategies of continuous quality improvement as one of the most promising new developments in health care:

Total quality management recommends itself for three main reasons. It is grounded in management strategies designed to *prevent quality problems* during the process of production, rather than simply measure them after they occur. It provides a fundamentally different review of the *relationship between quality and cost.* In industry it has proven that improvement in quality leads to lower cost by reducing waste, rework, and unnecessary complexity in the product process. Finally, it emphasizes the long-held and deeply ingrained principle in medicine of *continual learning* to improve care.

The long-term impact of *the new paradigm* on health care cannot yet be fully assessed, but its results to date have been promising.[11]

However, one thing that is not desirable as a result of continuous quality improvement initiatives is the defining of patient-care protocols as if patients were widgets or automobiles where agreed-upon manufacturing standards of quality guarantee good products. Human beings are enormously variable in their reactions to illness and their response to treatment, and physicians must realize that clinical quality improvement enables them to identify opportunities for organizing procedures and improve them in ways that make it easier to respond appropriately and effectively to individual patient needs.

As Dr. Cordy observes, "If for example, we find we really don't have to do as much blood work as we've been doing in order to get the information we need, then it simply makes sense to make the change in our practices. Not to do so would be a waste of time and resources, and cause unneeded discomfort for patients."

At St. Joseph's in a recent initial study of 105 consecutive repeat blood samples drawn from patients, it was found that approximately 65 per cent of them were unnecessary — and St. Joseph's is not that much different from most other Canadian hospitals.

Medical schools are also increasingly incorporating rigorous assessment of existing clinical data and literature as an integral part of physicians' training; as well, they are placing more emphasis on the physician's role as part of an interdisciplinary team. The issues of resource utilization — from rates of surgery and diagnostic tests to number of physician visits — have surged to the forefront of health care policy in the current environment of constraint.

"Eventually, whether we like it or not, external sources such as government are going to demand of us that we show them data that what we are doing is effective," says Dr. Cooper. "Physicians' practices are going to increasingly be under a microscope. The public expects it, government expects it, and most physicians now realize that the days of ever expanding resources for health care are gone and will not likely return. The real question is: Does what we do really make a difference and can we prove it?"

The public does not really recognize how variable the practices of physicians, let alone hospitals, are, and the implications of this for quality of care to individual patients, as well as the costs to taxpayers.

The dean of medicine at the University of Western Ontario, Dr. Robert McMurtry, observes that only 15 to 20 per cent of medical practice has ever been proven effective. This does not mean that much of the other

80 per cent is ineffective, but that we have no concrete basis upon which to judge the results of many treatment procedures.

Medicine has historically been based on the precept "Do no harm" — not "Do good," just "No harm." Physicians today are very aware that we are now at a point in history where it is imperative to focus on doing good and further, to prove it.

For physicians, the greatest positive potential of continuous quality improvement applied to clinical processes and patient programs is that they can use CQI tools and implementation strategies to take ownership of the process of change and bring about improvements from *within* medical practice that improve outcomes, rather than have to cope with externally imposed changes, which can only be conflictual. If hospitals become motivated during this decade and into the next to move toward total quality management, it will create hospitals that today's physicians only dream about.

4

The Hospital as a Learning Organization

The organizations that will truly excel in the future will be the organizations that discover how to tap people's commitment and capacity to learn at all levels in the organization.
— PETER SENGE, *THE FIFTH DISCIPLINE*

Total quality management will not just happen miraculously the moment hospital leaders decide to guide their institutions in that direction. Personally, this is the most difficult organizational change I have ever led. In the new order of health care that is emerging, hospitals must recognize that their enormous complexity can be turned from a difficult obstacle to a great strength. Every day, medical professionals in our hospitals have to be on top of all kinds of new and complex information. We are now at the point where medical knowledge literally doubles every five years. As well as being centres of the most up-to-date medical practices, today's hospitals are also environments where people learn to respond quickly to unexpected situations — from crises in the emergency department to patients experiencing complications during treatment to life-and-death-situations in the operating room.

Hospitals are organizations where highly developed skills and constant learning should be the order of the day. Recent developments in organizational and educational thinking are now urging a new approach to learning that will be necessary for business, industry, and the service sector to survive in future. In order to be capable of working in a health care system that is so rapidly changing and evolving, health care staff require new skills that go beyond their own medical or professional disciplines. They need to learn how to function effectively in dramatically changing organizations and environments.

Health care organizations, along with business and industry, must create environments conducive to continuous learning, becoming what Peter Senge in his provocative book *The Fifth Discipline* calls "the learning organization." The concept of continuous or lifelong learning for *individuals* has gained a good level of acceptance in educational institutions and in a few workplaces today. But the idea of a learning *organiza-tion*, the company or hospital in its entirety a learner, ventures into uncharted territory. Yet this has been identified as an unquestionable requirement for future organizational survival. According to *Fortune* magazine, the most successful organization of the 1990s and beyond will be "something called a learning organization, a consummately adaptive enterprise."[1]

THE PRINCIPLE OF CREATIVE TENSION

If a large organization is going to create for itself a pervasive learning environment that will carry it successfully into the future, two things are necessary: first, a vision of what the organization would like to be, and second, an accurate reading of things as they are now. Senge calls this difference the "principle of creative tension." When individuals and groups learn how to work with the energy (tension) created by this difference, they can achieve significant and long-lasting transformation. This principle represents a subtle, yet dramatic departure from the familiar and pervasive problem-solving orientation of how many contemporary organizations look at problems.

Senge's colleague Robert Fritz, who has done some important contemporary work in the area of human creativity and upon whose theories Senge draws, has observed that when we are in a problem-solving orientation, the focus is on making something, namely the problem, go away. For example, if for some reason there is frequently a delay in getting a patient admitted to a certain hospital floor with the proper tests and other necessary information, then the staff involved might meet to come up with strategies to ensure the delay doesn't happen. If they are successful, they will have made the problem go away and will naturally return to other problems.

While there is certainly nothing wrong with achieving this immediate result, it is only long-term results, *the creation of a new reality*, that will ultimately make the difference. To see desired long-term results, in this case perhaps effective changes to testing and admitting processes throughout the hospital, a different mind-set is needed. St. Joseph's has created a vision of eventually having no admitting department. Patients will arrive in the nursing unit with all information related to their case already available; in fact, patients will arrive on the day they are scheduled for surgery. The vision is to ensure anticipated discharge is reorganized to best benefit the patients (customers), that is, from the families' and patients' points of view.

Solving problems without the context of a larger vision of what you want to accomplish, actually may take energy *away* from the impetus to change rather than adding energy *to* it, because there is a sense of relief or complacency that sets in after a problem is "solved." This, observes Fritz, is why so many agendas for change fail — they simply lose their energy. A problem-solving mind-set results not in continuous improvement but in continuous oscillation between circumstances and the experience of either reacting or responding to those circumstances. The result is that the solutions do not last and people slowly, sometimes quickly, revert to the old pattern dictated by circumstances.[2] There is good evidence in all hospitals of this inability to maintain the gains, a situation that is frustrating to many.

The opposite state of affairs Fritz calls "the orientation of the creative," which allows a new "structure" to come into play — that of a creative, or structural, tension between where you are and where you want to be. In this orientation, problem-solving is transformed into the steps you need to take to bring about the desired result — the reality you wish to create. The energy and momentum within the orientation of the creative will guide both individuals and organizations naturally onto the path of continuous learning. The rate at which organizations learn may became the only sustainable source of competitive advantage.

No one can deny that the health care system and the health professionals who work within it are under considerable tension trying to respond adequately to rapid and complex medical and economic changes. There are two ways hospital senior management can become clearly aware of this tension. You can ask health care staff in any hospital what problems or barriers prevent them from doing their job the way they would like. Immediately you will hear stories of dissatisfaction, of things they know could be done better — "Dr. Smith's waiting room is too small and patients are standing in the hall"; "Whenever we order a special diet for a patient, it always takes at least a couple of days before we can get it"; or, "My staff are overworked because there's just not enough of us, and it bothers us that some patients have to be turned away."

Or you can try the other awareness strategy — create a vision that is so good, so positive, you want to be there instead of where you are. Imagining what *could* be is guaranteed to make you discontent with what *is*.

Ask: "If you were the patient, what would make this the best possible experience? What could we as providers do to organize our behaviour and practices to make it so?" But most effective of all, drawing on the principle of creative tension, align the two — the reality and the dream. Allow the tension between current reality and the vision of the future to become the bridge for creating total quality. The experience of tension from a state of crisis alone cannot do it. The tension needs, as Senge puts it, "a place to go," a vision of the future. A transformational leader has the capability to shift the focus from problem-solving to creating new visions that challenge the prevailing mental models," write A. Diane Moeller and Kathryn Johnson, two leading health care administrators in the U.S. "Creating organizational purpose is not enough. Leaders must promote a shared vision of the future that permeates throughout the organization and provides the guiding focus for current and future activities."3

That vision does not mean more resources, but a better use of them. Existing resources are realigned to achieve the vision. To prepare St. Joseph's Health Centre for total quality management, senior management leaders initiated both aspects of the principle of creative tension — an exploration of where things were at, and the creation of a quality vision for the future of the Health centre in the next decade and beyond.

TAKING THE PULSE OF ST. JOSEPH'S

When I arrived at St. Joseph's in late 1988, there were some important features of the culture that became apparent to me early on. If one looks at any organization that is to undergo major change, at least two important dimensions of that organization come into play.

First, there is the breadth of its values and commitment. There was no question that St. Joseph's possessed significant strengths in this dimension. Second, an organization needs certain types of specific knowledge and skills to get it where it needs to be in the current environment.

These latter characteristics were not as strong and would require some effort. But quite frankly, I prefer a health care organization with strong patient- and people-oriented values as its strengths because it is far easier (in relative terms) to develop new skills and create new knowledge than it will ever be to develop good positive and ethical values, which are lacking in some organizations.

In 1989, we used an evaluation tool to assess what our current organizational culture was like — the shared beliefs and values guiding the behaviour of hospital managers. Using the Organization Culture Inventory, a research tool available through Human Synergistics Inc., we surveyed 90 managers about their perceptions of organizational norms and expectations within the hospital. The Organizational Culture Inventory defines twelve types of organizational culture — affiliative, humanistic-helpful, approval, conventional, dependence, avoidance, oppositional, power, competitive, competence/perfectionistic, achievement, and self-actualization.

The results revealed that many members of the Health Centre's management staff were functioning in styles that tended toward an authoritarian emphasis on roles and functions; as well, they obtained high scores on the avoidance-culture scale — hoping problems will go away. When repeated a year later with 24 managers after a significant effort was made to challenge the managers to change, the inventory provided us with encouraging news — St. Joseph's management culture was starting to shift more toward an affiliative, humanistic-helpful, self-actualization style. In 1993 we will repeat the Organizational Culture Inventory by sampling managers, physicians, and CQI teams.

In the fall of 1991, all 3,200 hospital staff and the more than 300 physicians at the Health Centre were asked to participate in a Quality Climate Survey, an instrument developed by 3M Canada, to measure staff perceptions in 10 areas: organization, management support, communications, teamwork, problem-solving, reward and recognition, measurement, customer orientation, training, and general concerns. The survey yielded a 60 per cent response rate from the staff and 50 per cent from the physicians.

The physicians' ratings and assessment of the organization were virtually the same as the rest of the staff's. Thus the opportunities and needs for change had clear similarities across the hospital. A key finding was that while 68 per cent of respondents felt that employees would respond openly to the survey, only 28 per cent believed management would act on the results, an indicator that if continuous quality improvement was to be

ORGANIZATIONAL CLIMATE SURVEY
General Response

Strongly Agree/Agree 68%

Don't Know 10%

Strongly Disagree/
Disagree 7%

Neither 15%

Q86. I feel employees will respond openly to this survey

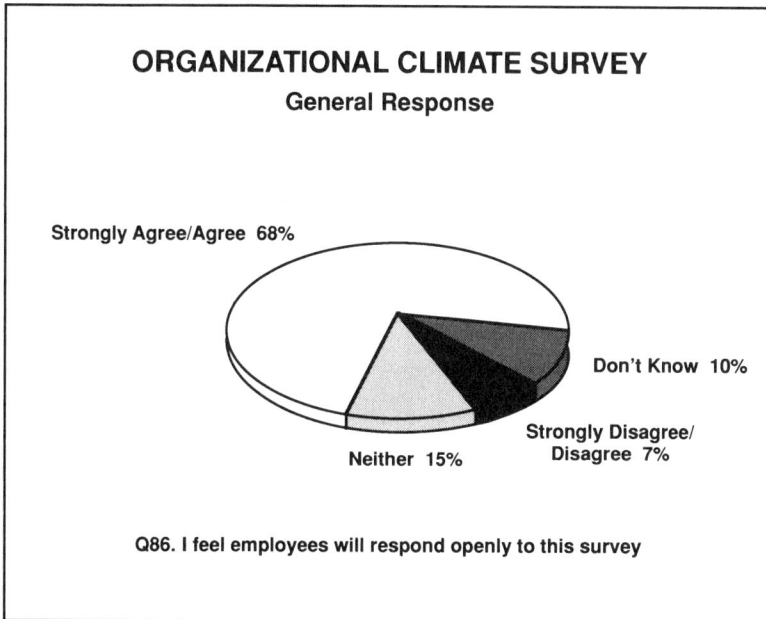

successful, senior management's involvement would have to be far more visible and concrete.

The staff identified one of St. Joseph's greatest strengths as its team-work, with 72 per cent expressing high satisfaction with it. We planned to take advantage of this strength. A key opportunity for improvement the survey identified was the need for more systematic and clearly defined strategies for reward and recognition. Physicians also indicated dissatisfaction with how they were rewarded and recognized for doing high-quality work at the Health Centre and said they wanted clearer communication with the administration.

The 1991 Quality Climate Survey provided good base-line information on staff's and physicians' perceptions of the hospital at that time. This survey, which we will repeat in 1993 and 1995, is an important way to measure the inroads and improvements being accomplished by the hospital's ever-growing focus on total quality management.

St. Joseph's Health Centre also commissioned the Angus Reid Group to survey external customers — 500 members of the general public in London, two-thirds of whom at one time or another had been patients at St. Joseph's. The hospital was rated "good" to "very good" in all areas.

ORGANIZATIONAL CLIMATE SURVEY
Work Group

Strongly Agree/Agree 72%

Don't Know 1%

Strongly Disagree/
Disagree 13%

Neither 14%

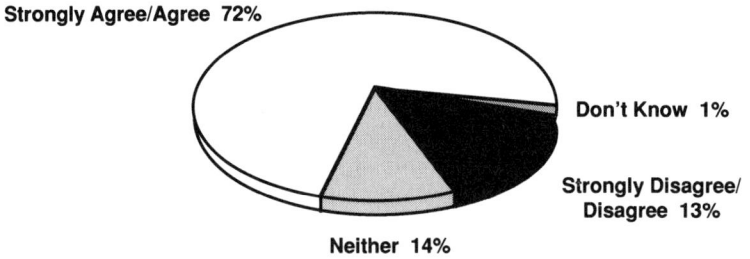

Q41. Considering everything, I am satisfied with the teamwork in my group

ORGANIZATIONAL CLIMATE SURVEY
General Response

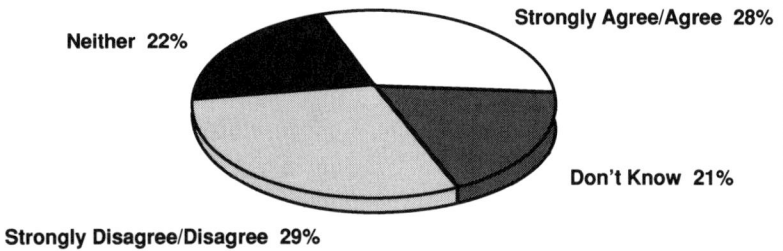

Neither 22%

Strongly Agree/Agree 28%

Don't Know 21%

Strongly Disagree/Disagree 29%

Q87. I feel that senior management will act upon the results of the survey

When asked which hospital they would choose to be admitted to, 38 per cent responded "St. Joseph's," compared to 33 and 22 per cent for the other two local acute-care hospitals.

One of the most important findings in light of St. Joseph's commitment to undertake total quality management was that members of the general public rated "having a reputation for treating patients with care and compassion" as the most important criteria for selecting a hospital (tied with "having an excellent emergency department"). It was significant that respondents rated St. Joseph's the highest in the care-and-compassion category among the three London acute-care hospitals.

This study was not intended to be critical of others but to assess what the community thought of us and to identify our opportunities for improvement. St. Joseph's emergency department was not rated as well as one of the other London acute-care hospitals. This improvement opportunity was grasped by Dr. David Taylor, chief of emergency services; Ann Croft, the nurse manager; and emergency room staff. They have since made important strides in improving emergency services at St. Joseph's — a project highlighted in Chapter Five.

FORMULATING A VISION STATEMENT

While these surveys were conducted and their results tabulated, the crucial future-oriented aspect in fostering a learning organization receptive to total quality management was also in process at the Health Centre — creating our vision of the future in the form of a statement that would be shared throughout the entire organization.

A vision statement is different from a mission statement. A mission statement outlines what the organization is, and its purpose. Organizational consultant Ian Percy observes that service organizations, particularly hospitals and nonprofit community agencies, have traditionally spent a lot of time crafting mission statements, which he describes as "a lot of nice words and good intentions that people just put on the back burner as they go about their business. After a while, they just don't get excited about them anymore."

A vision statement, on the other hand, paints a picture of where you want to go. At St. Joseph's we saw our vision as grounded within our mission. This mission speaks of the tradition of compassionate care of the sick, of the sacredness and dignity of human life, and of excellence in everything we do: patient care, teaching, and research. All hospitals, whether their origins are religious or secular, are grounded in positive values and principles out of which their future visions can be created.

As senior management became more comfortable with the concepts of total quality management, we began to visualize what our future would look like as a hospital where continuous quality improvement would be pervasive throughout every patient-care program or care process, whether on-site or off. Our objective became to develop a picture of what St. Joseph's would be in five to seven years while allowing for further evolution, further visioning, as we transformed. Within the context of TQM, our vision expresses the direction and characteristics of the Health Centre as we commit ourselves to the achievement of total quality. The vision plays a central role in helping us position our customers' expectations of us and the expectations staff members have of each other.

At the May 1991 three-day retreat on total quality management (see Chapter Two), the senior management team began to generate ideas about the vision and to formulate the criteria of an effective vision statement: that it should be developed by leaders within the organization, supported by Health Centre teams, and shared by the community. Other key criteria were that the vision would inspire the Health Centre to move forward, be framed in a comprehensive systems context, convey a positive tone, be easily recalled, and fit with the hospital's expressed mission, which is grounded in its history.

The next crucial step was to define a process for involving staff, because a vision created solely by management would not adequately reflect the hopes, dreams, and imagination of St. Joseph's as a whole. Staff in 51 areas watched a video featuring futurist Joel Barker, entitled *The Power of Vision*. To create a shared vision they were then asked to reflect on what they imagined the Health Centre should be like in the future, and to submit key statements and phrases that captured the quality and content of our vision of the future. In addition to staff, the Medical Advisory Committee, the Health Centre board, the Quality of Work Life Committee, St. Mary's Long-Term Care task force, and participants of an "Introduction to CQI" workshop were all asked for feedback on a first draft of our vision statement.

The result, after several drafts and several weeks of dialogue throughout the hospital, was a three-paragraph vision statement born of the culture and values of St. Joseph's Health Centre as a whole and shared by the community. Concurrent with creating a vision statement, the hospital also produced a video, *Living the Vision,* to be shared among staff, with other hospitals, and with the outside community. Our Vision Statement reads:

Caring Together:
We are committed to being an outstanding academic health centre that challenges everyone to work together to surpass expectations. We create an environment where teamwork and leadership enable compassion and excellence to prevail.

Improving Quality:
Inspired by our traditions and guided by our values, we will use our resources wisely, continuously improving the quality of life and health of those we serve and the processes of delivering care.

Serving Our Communities:
We will create an exceptional work environment for caring, learning, innovation, research and scientific inquiry in partnership with other health care providers to anticipate and meet the diverse needs of our communities.

We had a good idea of where we were and a vision of where we would like to be. But while the process of taking our pulse and forging the dream of our future was taking place, other initiatives were being developed and implemented as well. One of the great difficulties with telling the story of how St. Joseph's Health Centre began the shift from the old paradigm of department-based structures and a problem-filled health care system to a culture of cross-functional teams and problems perceived as the basis for new vision and future-oriented strategies, is that the process is not linear. It is not a straight road from point A to point B. Even as I write this, the vision we created seems to some, myself included, ironically short-sighted after only eighteen months, and in the months and years to come St. Joseph's Health Centre will create yet further-reaching visions to capture the dynamic transformation taking place throughout the institution.

For example, from the articulation of the vision has evolved a further refinement in the expression of the values St. Joseph's Health Centre will carry throughout all the dramatic changes in health care and well into the next century. The values clarification task force was formed under the leadership of Quality Council. The task force's goal was to articulate the corporate values which would guide the Health Centre in decision-making. The task force extracted value statements from a variety of documents including data gathered during the development of the vision statement, comments from the quality climate survey, the reward and recognition focus groups, evaluations from CQI workshops, strategic planning, mission statement, and the bioethics decision-making process.

From these documents it virtually seemed like hundreds of values emerged, and so, using an affinity diagram, major themes and naturally related ideas were placed together. Grouping ideas, discerning the meaning of words, probing, refining, and crafting a statement — all this was a thoughtful and often soul-searching experience. In the end, we created a draft values statement and tested it by asking "What does this say to you . . . what is your first reaction to hearing this statement?" Staff responses included: "It gives me a warm feeling," friendly," "spiritual," and "inspirational." Some staff also cautioned us, "Let's not put these words on the wall, but rather internalize them."

Our values statement reads as follows:

Above all else . . .
A Compassionate Spirit
Caring and Serving with Respect
Collaborating Creatively
Using Resources Wisely
Pursuing Knowledge Every Day
Trusting One Another
Giving Our Best

Although I often use the term "pathway" in reference to total quality management, a better term might be "tapestry" into which many colours, textures, and images are woven to create a whole. And so, while assessing our hospital's climate and creating our future vision, we also developed a comprehensive educational strategy that would initiate and maintain processes of TQM and CQI. What we wanted was an approach to education that emphasized not the role of the teacher per se, but the process of learning. More than anything else, the future of our industries, businesses, hospitals, and other key societal institutions will depend on people who do not just master knowledge, but rather continually apply learning processes to the accomplishment of both personal and organizational goals.

VALUES CLARIFICATION PROCESS

Objective established

↓

Task Force * formed
    * Task Force formed:
- 2 Vice Presidents
- 2 Directors
- 2 Managers
- Assistant to President
- Ad Hoc - Consultant

↓

Documents ** reviewed
    **Documents reviewed:
- Mission Statement
- Vision Statement input
- Quality Climate Survey results
- Reward and Recognition
- Focus Groups
- CQI Training Evaluations
- Bioethical Decision Making Process
- Vision Statement - Patient Services
- Strategic Plan
- Patient Comment Cards

↓

Ideas clustered using affinity program

↓

Key values identified

↓

Statement crafted

↓

Feedback† solicited
    † Feedback solicited from:
- Management Committee
- Bioethics Education Committee
- Selected managers and staff from education, nursing, human resources
- Executive of Board

↓

Statement revised by Task Force

↓

Completed statement presented to Board

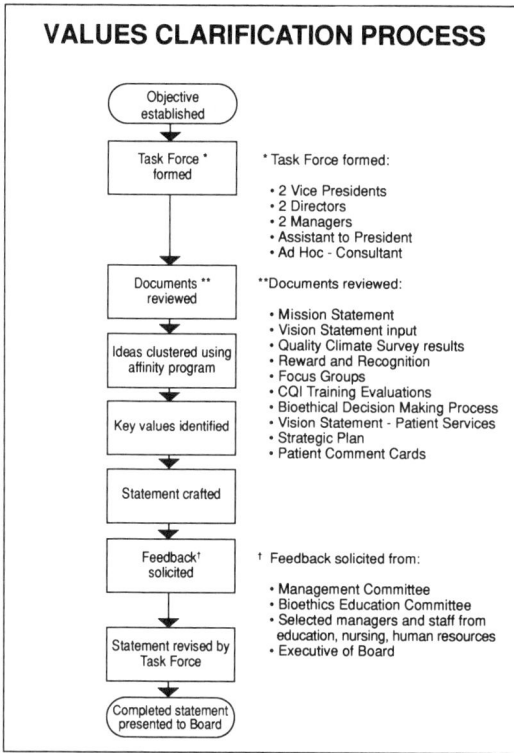

As we create this new thinking about learning, I realize as I never have before how profoundly important this major shift is; how, by investing in that resource we verbalize as most important, our people have become far more real and personal to me and many others in leadership roles at St. Joseph's. It is the challenge of the decade — to commit the organization to those we serve by creating a powerful workforce capable of energizing themselves and others to achieve the vision of the organization.

THE NEW ERA OF "KNOWLEDGE WORKERS"

Peter Drucker has written cogently of the role of knowledge and learning in what he defines as the fundamental shift from the concept of "Western" history and civilization to the concepts of "world history" and "world civilization." He writes: "In this society, knowledge is *the* primary resource for individuals and for the economy overall. Land, labour, and capital — the economist's traditional factors of production — do not disappear, but they become secondary. They can be obtained, and obtained easily, provided there is specialized knowledge. At the same time, however, specialized knowledge by itself produces nothing. It can become productive only when it is integrated into a task. And that is why the knowledge society is also a society of organizations: the purpose and function of every organization, business and non-business alike, is the integration of specialized knowledges into a common task."4

Of all philosophies and practices currently dealing with this challenge of integrating such "specialized knowledge" into a common vision, total quality management holds the most promise, because it is a means of co-ordinating many complex factors and producing data to measure the extent of positive change. Drucker observes that ideas of continuous quality improvement have, in fact, roots far back in history, in the excellence achieved by those who have always worked within the creative orientation.

The successful organization of the future, writes Drucker, "must devote itself to creating the new . . . The first is continuing improvement of everything the organization does, the process the Japanese call *kaizen*. Every artist throughout history has practised *kaizen*, or organized, continuous self-improvement. But so far only the Japanese — perhaps because of their Zen tradition — have embodied it in the daily life and work of their business organizations . . . The aim of *kaizen* is to improve a product or service so that it becomes a truly different product or service in two or three years' time."5

The orientation of *kaizen* depends in large part on the development of the "knowledge worker" within organizations. People are the greatest asset of any TQM initiative, and it is the synergy of their learning, skills, and talents that is the spirit of total quality.

"Because the modern organization consists of knowledge specialists," Drucker observes, "it has to be an organization of equals, or colleagues and associates. No knowledge ranks higher than another; each is judged by its contribution to the common task rather than by any inherent superiority or inferiority. Therefore, the modern organization cannot be an organization of boss and subordinate. It must be organized as a team."6

This is a tall order for a hospital, where role definition frequently takes the form of "turfism," and where, as I have mentioned earlier, the environment is organized more along separate departmental lines rather than in cross-functional relationships. The shift toward shared decision-making and self-directed teams is more than just total quality management jargon; it is the heart of total quality management. At St. Joseph's, for example, we have one self-directed team and other groups considering it. New ideas, and people given more scope, will produce new and better approaches resulting in some of the solutions or indicators of solutions for our organization and other ones.

IN-HOSPITAL EDUCATION: A NEW DIRECTION

Total quality management in health care relies not only upon learning and using a new set of tools and strategies to enable continuous quality improvement to take hold in the hospital, but also, and more fundamentally, upon the development among health professionals and hospital support staff of a whole new way of thinking. But having said this, we need to know how to create this new mind-set — how to lay the groundwork for the vision and to translate it into action.

The way is simple but not easy, for it involves the commitment of enormous resources of time, talents, and energies by staff. The philosophy, values, and practices of TQM must be *learned* by a critical mass of people, that is, a large enough group of people to effectively transform the organizational culture and then maintain the momentum of CQI, consistently focusing on the system's end purpose — to serve patients and their families. (Some organizational experts estimate that 30 to 40 per cent of the workforce in an organization constitutes critical mass, which results in the energy moving toward positive change becoming greater than the energy mitigating against it. Personally, I think the percentage is higher than that, perhaps two-thirds or more of individuals committed to change within an organization.)

In many of the current articles and books on total quality management in both business/industry and health care, education and training make up one of the key support systems that must be in place for an organization to shift to the values and practices of TQM. I would take this a step further and say that education and training, that is, learning, are *fundamental* to the success of total quality management, indeed to the success of organizations as a whole. Staff must feel secure in their understanding of the concepts and techniques of total quality management, and be continually supported in their quest for information that will help them achieve quality goals.

In the context of any large, complex organization such as a hospital, the concept of continuous learning has as much to do with *doing* as it does with attending educational sessions designed specifically to address concepts of total quality management. Part of the dynamic of TQM is that doing and learning take place simultaneously, even though individuals may not yet feel comfortable with the new tools of change they are being asked to work with. In the quality arena, there is no way you can first know everything that needs to be done and then begin to create quality in all you do. Both are done together.

That is why we began four demonstration projects at approximately the same time we launched the TQM education and training. In the next several pages, I will be focusing on this education and training process, and in the following chapter you will read about the demonstration projects and other "from learning to action" strategies.

In order to meet the challenge of moving the hospital toward total quality management, our educational services department began the process, which is still ongoing, of developing its leading role in the transformation of the hospital. This has entailed a shift in the model of teaching and learning, one that reflects not only the demands of total quality management but the future direction of educational systems in general.

The educational system many adults today have grown up with was didactic, one that focused on the authority of the teacher, a fixed content that had to be covered, "right" answers, and a passive learning style (teacher talks, student listens). In many workplaces, hospitals included, this same system extends itself into the dominant model of management where managing is accomplished largely by policy and procedure, individual (not team) performance is the main focus, and the ability to think, reflect, and innovate is discouraged, and in some cases actively stifled.

The kind of innovation, risk-taking, and creativity inherent in total quality management means that this old paradigm of education must give way to a model of education that centres on the learner. Learner-centred (customer-focused) education has come to be identified as the most effective way to teach adults, but also increasingly is making inroads into the classrooms of elementary and secondary schools searching for ways to better prepare students for the complexities and challenges of the adult world. In hospitals, where the learning tasks are numerous and demanding, educational services departments have over the years steadily evolved toward this learner-centred approach to training and professional development. In many hospitals, there is a good fit between the already existing commitment to adult education values and the values that drive organizational change toward total quality management.

In a learner-centred system, teaching is based on a participant's knowledge and experience, as well as on his or her current needs and goals. From the management perspective, the organization builds on workers' knowledge of work systems at all organizational levels to design and negotiate change in both systems and processes. In other words, the people best qualified to make positive changes are the ones doing the work. In the new paradigm of total quality management, organizations create a safe and rewarding climate for learning and dialogue, an environment where coaching toward continuous growth and improvement, rather than criticism for shortcomings, is the norm. As Peter Senge advocates, learning and dialogue go far beyond the model of simply encouraging discussion, during which ideas may be shared, but not assimilated or acted upon.

Many hospitals have an educational services department that provides professional development opportunities and updating for staff members as part of the mandate to keep them current about new developments in organizational and health care practices. Today, hospitals' educational services departments play an indispensable role in helping cope with the current knowledge explosion within health care.

In the hospital as a learning organization, effective educators (initially from the educational services department, but eventually involving staff from other areas) spearhead training that leads toward the goal that managers themselves will gain the skills to build strong work teams. They will give effective support to cross-functional teams involved in system improvement projects. Senge talks about "generative learning" — learning as a self-directed, empowering process leading to increasing momentum for innovation and continuous improvement. Not only do processes of continuous quality improvement support such generative learning, but they provide tools of measurement and data gathering that enable individuals and teams to assess outcomes accurately.

The learner-centred education model, so crucial to the success of total quality management in health institutions, is not restricted exclusively to staff training *within* hospitals, however. It can also be a dynamic strategy in creating effective patient-education programs. Many hospitals have developed innovative learner-centred, patient-focused education programs, and these, too, can be incorporated into the TQM focus in terms of gathering data to assess the effectiveness and levels of satisfaction with patient education. The Western Ontario Provincial Lithotripsy Program, for example, modified its patient-education materials by including a short fact sheet in its patient-education brochure in response to finding out through a patient-satisfaction questionnaire that seven per cent of patients expressed considerable anxiety about not having been informed about the possibility of having a stent inserted. (A stent is a small tube inserted in the urinary tract prior to having a kidney stone crushed or removed. It ensures appropriate bladder drainage and helps pass stone fragments.) Since as many as 50 per cent of kidney stone patients have stents and about 25 per cent of those who arrive at the unit without stents need to have them inserted, the lithotripsy clinical staff realized that the seven per cent of patients who brought up the issue likely represented a more widely held patient concern.

The use of CQI strategies in designing patient education and health promotion programs is a promising new direction for health care. I discuss this issue further in Chapter Five, but for now I want to come back to the focus on the role of education and training in implementing TQM. Our training materials in continuous quality improvement did not spring full-blown into well-organized presentations and workshops, but were the result of careful groundwork, design, and many long hours.

PREPARING TO LEARN TOTAL QUALITY MANAGEMENT
When I assumed the position of president and CEO, the Health Centre's educational services department already possessed many positive strengths in the area of learner-centred training. In 1987, for example, peers teaching peers became a key methodology for in-hospital nursing training through a preceptorship model which involved nursing staff in leadership and teaching roles, and a model of collegiality in the delivery of patient care throughout the health centre. Hence, a simple key of learning applied: use the existing strengths of the organization.

During the period shortly after my arrival, when I and other members of senior management were making early explorations into the potential of total quality management for St. Joseph's, we asked educational services to provide us with some training in such areas as team-building, problem-solving skills, and leadership development. These were, and still are, crucial to moving us forward.

3M Canada handed over its industrial material "Managing Total Quality" for our revision early in 1990. At that point, St. Joseph's educational services department, particularly department manager Peggy Roffey, began the massive revision process necessary to "translate" the industrial model to health care. Fortuitously, Roffey was a candidate for a Ph.D. in English — an enormous benefit to us, given the task. "Customer" had to be understood in terms of patients, physicians, and internal staff. "Zero defects" had to be reframed as the achievement of appropriate treatment protocols that would ideally be without defect, but that also would account for the human variability of patients who respond to treatment as individuals, and so forth.

The customization of the 3M materials became more complex when 3M's materials from the United States had to be amalgamated with the adaptation already begun by St. Joseph's. In order not to delay the piloting in July 1991 of the learning materials at St. Joseph's, we made use primarily of the American materials. Our own revisions up to that point were available for use only in part. By November 1991, the St. Joseph's-U.S. amalgamated version was complete and subsequently implemented as the core curriculum of CQI training designed specifically for health care.

The pilot workshop of July 1991, involving managers as well as facilitators who had been selected to assist continuous quality projects (see Chapter Five), took place over a five-day period. The response to this program, entitled "Introduction to CQI," was enthusiastic. There was a sense of excitement as staff began to realize that CQI strategies could put a more positive face on many of the challenges confronting health care workers and the health care system in general.

One staff member evaluating the pilot workshop said, "I learned, gathered new information, gained many great things from a group of people I may not otherwise have had close access to." Said another, "The energy and enthusiasm generated will be a valuable asset to St. Joseph's in terms of launching the process and communicating the philosophy to other employees."

Workshop participants saw difficulties in fully adapting the industrial concepts to a health care setting. The sheer volume of information made it difficult to digest, as did the anticipated problems in communicating not just the concepts of total quality management but also in making changes throughout the Health Centre. "I certainly understand CQI now, but do not feel able to deliver," wrote one participant in her evaluation. The participants also felt that the five days required out of their busy schedules were far too much, an observation that led to reducing "Introduction to CQI" to three days.

In the fall of 1991, we began the process of introducing CQI training to management groups and other key individuals throughout the hospital. A sense of energy and excitement began to build among staff who increasingly were drawn to the realization that "finding a better way" could be more than a potential — it could be a reality. But the training also uncovered other important questions.

Questions such as, "Why do we need to do this anyway — isn't this just another management fad?" or, "What happens when a team comes up with a solution through a CQI project and a manager vetos it?" often came up during the workshop sessions, or were addressed to me during "hot seat" sessions at the conclusion of workshops, or at informally structured meetings with staff groups. These questions created important dialogue and, according to the staff, often left them inspired when they realized that they themselves could address these issues.

The education model adopted by St. Joseph's Health Centre is congruent with the concept of a learning organization, which must always adapt to new realities and always be open to questioning. During the education and training sessions, as well as in working on specific CQI projects, staff are encouraged to view the uncertainties they experience (largely due to TQM being unknown in many workplaces) as a learning challenge for growth and development. In the creative orientation, Robert Fritz has observed, there are no mistakes, no "wrong" ways, only opportunities for learning, the results of which you continually measure against the vision you wish to achieve. To paraphrase American organizational expert Leland Kaiser, there is not one way but an infinite number of ways of doing things.

Who Gets What Training?

We had decided that the total quality management roll-out of education and training processes would draw primarily upon the internal resources of time and talent at St. Joseph's. To do this, we chose what is known as a "cascade" model for teaching continuous quality improvement throughout the organization. The teaching team mobilized specifically for education and training in total quality management consisted of the educational services manager, three staff educators, two "seconded" managers, the director of total quality management, and senior management — including the president and five vice-presidents. This combination of hospital staff to deliver the training programs is a crucial aspect of modelling the participatory, shared vision of total quality management, in that a key portion of the learning and dialogue during the three days is facilitated not by educational services staff, but by the quality director, the five vice-presidents, and the president. Physicians, the director of personnel, and various department managers and team leaders also participated in the teaching/learning dialogue over the three days.

The concept of a cascade model of education is that the initial training given to managers is then "cascaded" down into the organization through managers and directors who teach their own front-line staff. After the pilot "Introduction to CQI" workshop had been modified from five days to three, educational services then began offering the program at approximately monthly intervals for members of the Quality of Work Life Committee, facilitators, union leaders, managers, directors, and project team leaders. Other staff identified as likely to take a role in teaching continuous quality improvement were clinical nurse specialists, charge nurses, and other individuals in supervisory roles; these people also participated in "Introduction to CQI." By the end of 1992, approximately 200 staff from these groupings were trained, representing virtually all the management staff and many others (about half) who, as noted above, are key to this change process. "Introduction to CQI" provides in-depth exploration of the philosophy and components of continuous quality improvement, training in work process analysis, staff roles and responsibilities (including physicians'), the cost of quality, quality teams, support systems, the creation of a quality annual plan, developing vision and success statements, and an overview of the change process.

Participants come to the sessions having already read the material. The sessions are interactive, involving both small and large group exercises, as well as considerable dialogue and exchange of views. The focus on the customer, which in this case is the staff participating in the workshops, is evident in the encouragement of constant "kaizens" — written suggestions from staff for improvement of the sessions — the identification of individual expectations, and built-in flexibility in the agenda.

Each participant concludes the workshop with a personal action plan developed over the three days. This might be something such as "I'm going to ask my customers how they perceive some aspect of the service we are giving them," or, "I plan to read more articles on quality and Donald Berwick's book," or, "I'm going to discuss with my peers ideas for a possible improvement project we can begin right away."

Because a prime goal is to equip managers and directors to teach the concepts and practice of continuous quality improvement to front-line staff and because you learn best what you teach, on the last day of the introductory workshop, each participant teaches a ten-minute segment based on one of the course modules and receives feedback from peers. Joan Garrison, one of St. Joseph's Health Centre's nursing managers, who was seconded for six months to educational services, describes her feelings of first being confronted with the challenge of teaching continuous quality improvement to other staff.

"We had heard that this program called 'continuous quality improvement' was coming, and when we were presented with the task of participating in management-led cascade training, lots of us had initial feelings of frustration and anxiety. Often the first thing that came to mind was 'I'm not a teacher or a public speaker,' or, 'How am I supposed to do this within the existing budget?' or, 'Why should I spend fifteen minutes coaching someone to make a decision I normally would make in three minutes?'" recalls Garrison.

Even the assurance that managers and directors would have several months to complete the eight hours of teaching the program, entitled "Your Role in Quality," to front-line staff was small comfort in light of the wider significance of this challenge. "As managers we were accustomed to managing, taking responsibility for our departments and the decision-making procedures there. With continuous quality improvement, it was not just a matter of teaching the material, it was the realization that when staff put this material into action, our management roles are challenged. CQI models a changing perspective from managing to coaching — and it takes some time for managers to get used to seeing themselves as coaches and facilitators of work processes," Garrison observes. "It can be threatening to some."

A year into the training, Garrison noted that these anxieties were far less in evidence. "Now what I see is the enthusiasm of managers and an appreciation of how rewarding this shift in our relationship with staff can be. But it is not an easy task. There are a great deal of logistics involved, such as arranging release time for staff, scheduling training sessions. If your department is very large, this can get very complicated. And not all managers are comfortable working with a more self-directed staff. Needless to say, not all front-line staff are comfortable working this way either. They don't know yet if they can fully trust the process." Managers and directors are not thrown into this new teaching role cold after completing

"Introduction to CQI." They are offered a further two-day skills training workshop — "Teaching Your Role in Quality" — where they learn how to use the leaders' guide, how to schedule and facilitate sessions, and develop effective presentation skills. Structured into the workshop are opportunities to practise-teach 20-minute segments from the leaders' guide.

The next step in the cascade model is the actual roll-out to front-line staff in the format of an eight-hour orientation program called "Your Role in Quality." Thus far, staff have shown great flexibility in organizing this training to fit the needs of individual groups or departments. Some have opted for eight sessions of one hour. Others have scheduled the sessions in two-hour or four-hour blocks. "This is all part of being able to 'walk the talk' of quality in that we say to staff, 'Here are the materials,' and then each group has the flexibility and support to adapt the delivery of the program to their own needs," says Garrison.

By the time this book is published, I expect two-thirds, or 2,000, of front-line staff will have received the "Your Role in Quality" teaching. And by late 1993, virtually all staff will have had at least a basic orientation of eight hours in total quality management. "Your Role in Quality" is the program that brings TQM concepts most directly to busy front-line staff, and that sows the seeds of a new way of learning, doing, and working together that will lead to total quality. It is at this level that organizations discover whether or not they can succeed in translating concepts to practices.

"I had many misgivings at first," recalls Shelley Wood, an occupational therapist working in rehabilitation during the time she attended "Your Role in Quality." "We had heard rumours of an idealistic new program that would be coming to our department eventually, and I remember thinking this is probably going to mean a lot more work. I also thought if management has designed this new program, they probably don't realize that everything looks different in the trenches."

Then, after eight hours of training, Wood remembers being surprised that a wide variety of colleagues from other departments and disciplines were part of her learning group. "There were other OTs, physiotherapy aides, and therapists from other areas — people I didn't get to speak with much in the course of the average working day. And the interesting thing was that when we all got talking, we discovered we shared many of the same questions and misgivings. So you realize you're not alone in wondering what these changes will mean."

One particularly important insight she shared was that "many of the people sitting across from me I could begin to see as customers who expected a certain level of service from me, and in turn that I was their customer. I think it really increased our sense of accountability to each other."

Getting comfortable with the language of continuous quality improvement is also a challenge for many, Wood believes. Terms such as "customer" and "work processes" take getting used to, she says. "But you do begin to shift your thinking, and you find yourself thinking of ways to improve things. It can be a small change — such as when we decided to alter what we felt was an awkward discharge form to make it fit our needs better.

"Or continuous quality improvement can lead you to bigger changes. For example, in our rehabilitation area, we had what we thought was an excellent support group for stroke patients. We had become aware that participation in the group was waning, but we didn't know why. And so we used the CQI approach and surveyed these patients — our customers. What we discovered was that they preferred extra therapy sessions or to receive more support one on one than to attend groups. So here we were putting resources into a program our patients said was not benefiting them.

"This, I think, is the potential of CQI — it will help us identify what works and what doesn't. Actually stopping something that's not effective is new to us in health care," she concludes.

As more staff members encounter the "Your Role in Quality" program or hear about it from colleagues, many are now entering education and training sessions with a far higher level of awareness than was previously the case. Some may already be participating on CQI teams.

Consistent with the widening of hospital education and training for total quality management within the context of creating a learning organization, other learning opportunities support the achievement of a culture of total quality management. Facilitators, for example, take a further three-day workshop on work process analysis, and for team leaders there is a two-day session on team skills. More learning strategies in continuous quality improvement have been developed at St. Joseph's following a "just in time" teaching model: presentation skills, project management, consultation skills, customer service skills, creative problem-solving, and persuasive communication.

According to one of St. Joseph's staff educators, Jim Handyside, who has been working closely with team leaders and facilitators in teaching CQI methods and tools, the greatest learning challenge for many teams has not been the identification of processes that need improving ("That part is easy," Handyside says), but learning to ask the right questions that will lead them to an improvement methodology. "It is often a matter of knowing how to break the process down into measurable processes; for example, not why are there delays in getting patients from point A to point B, but what happens from the time a patient is at this point of the process until they reach the next one."

Another hurdle is the use of work process analysis tools, such as flow charts, bar graphs, and the collection of both quantitative and qualitative data (see Appendix 1 - Work Process Analysis tools). "The main objective here," says Handyside, "is to demystify these tools and show how they can be maps that allow teams to see where they are and to plan the direction of future improvements."

FUTURE CHALLENGES FOR THE LEARNING ORGANIZATION

The close, and indeed inextricable, link between total quality management and continuous quality improvement transforms organizations into what Peter Senge calls "learning laboratories." The learning model developed to deliver the education and training crucial to the achievement of total quality management eventually becomes self-perpetuating in the organization as staff are increasingly empowered to teach each other and learn from each other.

The role of educational services itself also evolves in a new direction. At St. Joseph's Health Centre, the educational services department will increasingly play a facilitating, coaching role as more hospital staff are enabled to participate actively in teaching and on project teams. Educational services will remain a key resource for the design and delivery of further training as needed. In addition, the department will devote more of its time to following up the results of the programs already delivered, and will also focus on the important role of learning in facilitating organizational development as a whole.

Through the involvement of health professionals from many different disciplines, as well as nonclinical staff in CQI training sessions, a solid foundation for hospital-wide change has become part of the organizational culture. I cannot emphasize enough that a strong priority accorded to education and learning is absolutely crucial to total quality management and to the creation of the learning organization as a whole. If a hospital is not prepared to invest in this crucial resource — its staff — and to devote a lot of time and resources developing a comprehensive, interactive, and flexible plan of education for total quality, it should not even begin the attempt to implement total quality management.

Some think they can get rid of those who have difficulty using the new skills. That may have worked in the past, but it is ultimately a sign of a short-sighted failing organization. People can be energized to learn, and learning is ultimately the responsibility of each individual. By walking the talk, senior leaders facilitate learning to occur at all levels, which will accordingly lead to behavioural changes fundamental to transformation. This will be the moment of truth for organizations to succeed.

My experience at St. Joseph's Health Centre confirms my belief in people. They are eager and excited to learn the possibilities of a better way for health care, most specifically for the patients they serve. In the next two chapters, I will talk about how we began translating this learning to action — through the formation of our total quality management organizational structure, the choice of the initial four demonstration projects, subsequent CQI teams and projects, and the development of further support systems, which add momentum to achieving a culture of total quality throughout the hospital.

5

The Quality Vision
at St. Joseph's

No single individual can operate today's complex organization. . . .
Leaders must possess the ability to choose and inspire a team of
people with diverse skills to accomplish the job.

A.D. MOELLER AND K. JOHNSON,

"SHIFTING THE PARADIGM FOR

HEALTH CARE LEADERSHIP"

Because total quality management is the beginning of a paradigm shift for hospitals, it requires a significant transformation of management structure — one that's dynamic and fluid rather than hierarchical, and inclusive of individuals collaborating across functions rather than defined exclusively by their departmentally based roles. Hierarchical management is in the twilight of its existence. No matter what sort of organization you are in, inherent in the model of total quality management is that it continually changes and evolves along with the increasing number of continuous quality improvement initiatives. This is the challenge we face at St. Joseph's Health Centre, and by all who venture down this road.

While we had already initiated key directions and strategies to move the Centre and heighten its awareness of the possibilities of TQI, the senior management May 1991 three-day retreat was one of several vital steps in getting started. So were our successful early attempts at total quality management through our lithotripsy program, which was designed with a strong customer focus, and our initial value improvement programs, which were aimed at clinical quality improvement processes.

THE BEGINNINGS OF A TQM ORGANIZATION STRUCTURE

The purpose of the May retreat was to begin to translate the philosophy and values of TQM into an action plan, realizing that we were neither on a short trip nor in a marathon, but rather on a continuous journey to places we had not yet imagined. We understood that a process of clear communication between senior leaders and middle managers and their front-line staff was crucial to achieve staff buy-in.

With this in mind, the senior management team designed a six-month action plan to launch total quality management effectively at St. Joseph's Health Centre. To convey clearly our collective role and commitment to total quality management, we first called ourselves the Quality Steering Committee. Our group structure has since evolved and is now called the Quality Council, made up of the CEO, the Health Centre's five vice-presidents, the chairman of the Medical Advisory Committee, and the director of total quality management; shortly, we will add the director of communications.

TOTAL QUALITY MANAGEMENT
SENIOR MANAGEMENT WORKSHOP

PRIORITIZED LIST OF IMPLEMENTATION ACTIONS

	Item	Action	Deadline
1.	Finalize Vision Statement	• Review and revise Draft #1	• May 29/91
2.	Prepare "elevator speech" to commun- incate what has been learned and next steps	• Practise during workshop	• May 23/91
3.	Clarify and communicate to managers the role of the CQI facilitator	• Draft letter detailing changes and arrange to meet with managers	• June 5/91
		• Develop education plan for facilitators and managers	
4.	Develop communication strategy for TQM	• Draft plan for Quality Council with a focus on defining terms through real examples	• June 24/91
5.	Link annual quality plan to strategic plan	• Draft a plan to reduce barriers to change	• June 24/91
6.	Develop measurement	• Incorporate both macro and micro evaluation measures	• June 24/91

The action plan included preparations for a pilot of the adapted 3M educational materials, the identification of results-oriented demonstration projects, the creation of a vision for the future (see Chapter Four), and the development of what we have come to call "elevator speeches" — speeches limited to 90 seconds during which the individual summarizes important consistent messages about total quality management. These brief elevator speeches are useful and informative teaching tools with busy health care staff.

Selection of Staff to Serve as Facilitators   Working on the principle that total quality management is best facilitated from within an organization using the skills of the people who work there, a next important step was to initiate a process to select continuous quality improvement facilitators. In June of 1991, St. Joseph's directors and managers were invited to an information-exchange session to review the selection criteria of facilitators and the expectations of both facilitators and managers.

Initially, 3M had recommended that staff members selected as facilitators would have 40 per cent of their time released to take on the facilitation responsibilities. Feedback from staff in front-line patient-care areas, as well as in many busy support areas, informed us this would not be feasible, and so we adjusted the plan to a 20-per-cent time commitment. Facilitator time would be focused on assisting teams, and managers would serve as teachers, allowing us to accommodate the reduced time. This was to be accomplished without the addition of extra staff — the Health Innovations grant from the provincial government only covered the development of the training materials and the implementation of evaluation strategies. The total quality management program itself was designed so as not to incur extra cost to the hospital budget — that is, taxpayer dollars.

Therefore, the understanding and support of managers was crucial, for if facilitators were chosen from their departments, they would have to do some departmental reorganization to allow the individuals time in their duties. Managers were asked to identify staff in their departments whom they felt showed leadership, teaching, and communication skills. Individuals were also encouraged to nominate themselves. At the end of the nomination period, we had 43 names from which were selected an initial 20.

The selection of facilitators from across the Health Centre who would work with future CQI teams was an extremely significant step in the shifting St. Joseph's Health Centre toward total quality management. It marked the beginnings of the transition from management-led change to wider staff involvement. We are now discovering that the investment and development required of facilitators may lead us to renegotiate our contract — so far, our facilitators are underutilized. The facilitators, while highly motivated, do not yet possess the confidence, nor have they fully internalized the concepts of work process analysis, given the limited opportunity to practise and the complexity of the processes to be analysed. Our team resource educators, Jim Handyside and Karen Shuttleworth, play a vital role in coaching facilitators through their initial team experience.

The Quality Council The six-month action plan laid the basis for St. Joseph's long-term total quality management implementation plan and embodied many of our key learnings as we shifted toward a new organizational culture. In particular, we came quickly to the realization that there is one aspect of management structure which must be "designed in" to the overall vision of total quality management from its beginnings within an organization. There must be a functional structure in place, one firmly anchored to the principle that senior leaders are visibly committed to total quality management and are willing to invest considerable time in its implementation.

At St. Joseph's, we created the Quality Council to provide this visible leadership. It works to ensure the implementation of innovative strategies across the hospital and co-ordinates the development of the annual operational quality plan. The council also plans, and helps identify and monitor, complex cross-functional opportunities with the continuous quality improvement teams. As well, each member of the Quality Council is responsible for portions of the teaching during CQI training.

The Quality Council, which meets weekly, frequently expands its membership to consult with representatives from educational services, communications, unions, physicians, and other hospital staff. Another group of staff makes up the TQM Implementation team. This group supports the Quality Council in coaching cross-functional clinical and nonclinical teams and refining the infrastructure at the Health Centre. The Medical Advisory Committee continues its existing link with the Audit Committee and is evolving that committee's role toward CQI. The Nursing Co-ordinating Council retains its connection with Nursing Quality Improvement. Each of St. Joseph's vice-presidents sponsors a number of teams departmentally and cross-functionally. In my case four years ago, I spent less than five per cent of my time thinking about quality. I now spend more than 50 per cent.

Perhaps as important to the senior management group as the immediacy of the issues surrounding total quality management, were the activities leading up to that time. My introduction to CQI had been in 1988, and it was evident that gaining early momentum by supporting others to attend conferences (at that time only available in the U.S.) was essential. Two of the vice-presidents and a few managers were sent to conferences in 1989 and 1990 which prepared them as credible change agents and helped initiate the process with the management group.

Surprised and impressed by the potential continuous quality improvement held, they were advocates from the beginning. Obviously, sending managers who already had credibility among their colleagues was crucial. As well, our "strategic think-ins" focused us on the magnitude and rapid pace of change descending upon the organization. There was great worry about where I was leading the Health Centre, but the several strategic think-ins between 1989-91, along with other strategies introduced to enable the senior management team to gear up for change, truly launched CQI with only minor adverse reactions.

Thus, the date we began implementing total quality management depends upon how you define the initiation stage. The one real mistake I made was getting ahead of the organization and talking to the media about our initiation of continuous quality improvement strategies. The reaction by one staff member was to dash off an angry letter to the *London Free Press*: "How dare the CEO suggest we don't deliver quality?" This incident caused the senior management team — and, humbly, me — to give more consideration to the pacing of CQI and to the communication of these changes externally. Again, we learned a lot about how language can be a stumbling block.

Two other decisions were critical. First, the requirement that senior management change. While a very difficult personal time for many, the kinds of changes we were looking for required thinking and vision that coincided with our future. Thus, within the first 18 months of my arrival, senior staff needed to determine their future based on what they saw and the phenomenal changes that were about to occur. Of the operating vice-presidents, five of six chose to leave, not necessarily because of the changes they saw happening. But it is clear in reviewing the history of leaders of organizational change that they often saw most of their senior staff leave.

The second critical decision was the hiring of a coordinator/director for total quality management — a coach for me and an intermediary to facilitate the multitude of changes which were surely on the horizon. We interviewed several people with good skills, but after much introspection by the committee, we decided to try to bring back Jane Parkinson, the former director of educational services who had left to join the Achieve Group, where she was an implementation consultant for several of their training programs included in their service quality system. We succeeded, and her many attributes and skills have helped make our TQM efforts successful. A nurse with a degree in Psychology, an educator with an M.Ed., and, most importantly, someone people feel comfortable talking with, she had high credibility with the staff and instantly met with positive reaction. Her consulting and teaching skills were helpful to the process changes and her ability to give me constructive feedback on my thinking and behaviour has helped me enormously.

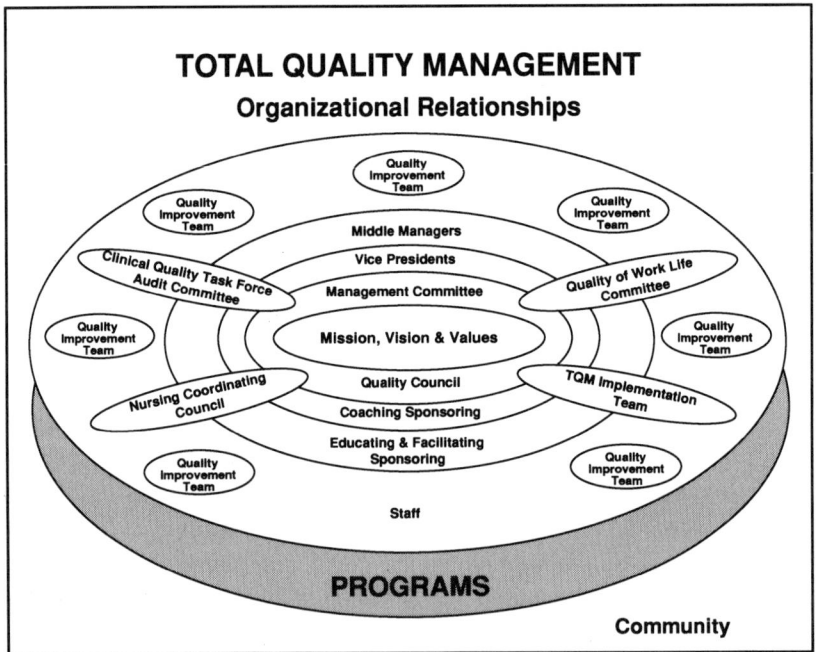

TOTAL QUALITY MANAGEMENT
Organizational Relationships

TQM DEPENDS ON THE ENERGY AND COMMITMENT OF TEAMS
The heart of total quality management at St. Joseph's Health Centre is the work of the continuous quality improvement teams. It is at this level that we see most clearly how TQM works to continuously improve care and service, and to increase patient and staff satisfaction. CQI teams are formed in order to study hospital processes from a *customer* perspective, find ways to build on existing strengths, eliminate redundancies or unnecessary steps, and to develop and implement continuous improvements.

THE CONTINUOUS QUALITY IMPROVEMENT PATHWAY

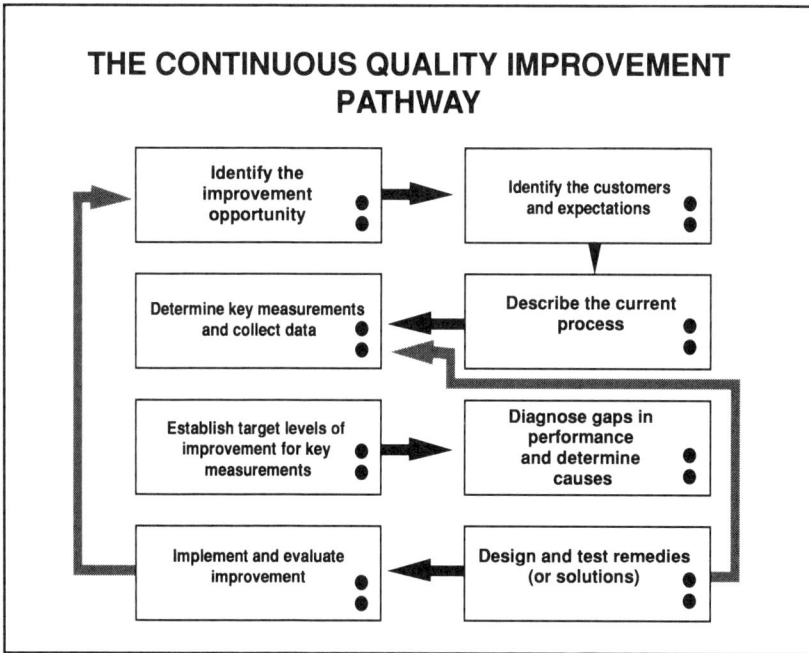

CQI projects can be organized in several ways — on an individual, departmental, divisional, or corporate basis. All projects take as their fundamental value the mission and vision statements of St. Joseph's Health Centre as a whole. Before describing the work of some of St. Joseph's CQI teams, I would first like to share with you how our teams are structured to allow them the maximum flexibility and support from the Health Centre as a whole.

The CQI *facilitator* helps to train and coach teams in applying CQI concepts and in using the tools and methods necessary for identifying an improvement process. The facilitator also assists the development of collaborative team skills. In most cases the facilitators are front-line staff from different areas who have committed 20 per cent of their time to improving team processes.

Each CQI team has a *team leader*. This is a staff person who is familiar with the process identified by the team for improvement and is chosen by his or her peers who are participating in the CQI project. The team leader heads the team meetings, facilitates the use of the improvement process, encourages effective group dynamics, and co-ordinates the team's activities with both department managers and the team facilitator.

It is from the *team members* themselves that the energy and commitment to improve care really begins to make a difference. From team members comes not only the analysis of work processes using tools and methods, but the design and implementation of the solutions. The team together takes ownership of the process, and each member has a stake in the project's implementation and monitoring of results.

There is another key role we created at St. Joseph's, one we find crucial to maintaining hospital-wide support for change. We call these individuals sponsors (we are in the process of renaming these individuals "mentors"). The sponsor, as the name suggests, supports teams by taking a mentor role and paves the way for the team to gather the resources it needs. Initially our sponsors were members of senior management, but as total quality management has begun to widen its base other key individuals are now ready to take on this role. As well as helping teams to see the process they are studying in the context of the whole system, to gather relevant information, and to help them communicate with the organization as a whole, another important aspect of the sponsor's role is to recognize a team's successes and make these successes known to others in the Health Centre.

None of the CQI teamwork could be accomplished without the commitment of *department managers*. Managers play a significant role in supporting the importance of CQI projects and also, along with the sponsors, assist teams to obtain needed resources.

We have taken considerable time at St. Joseph's Health Centre for the training of CQI team leaders and members in the methods and tools of continuous quality improvement, and in the development of team skills. As with any group process, CQI teams do not automatically become cohesive units working for improvement. Many members of the team have never worked together before — for example, physicians and nurses collaborating on a team with staff members from such areas as medical records or admitting. Frequently, role and function barriers must be broken down and people made to feel comfortable giving input to the team and having their participation and viewpoints appreciated.

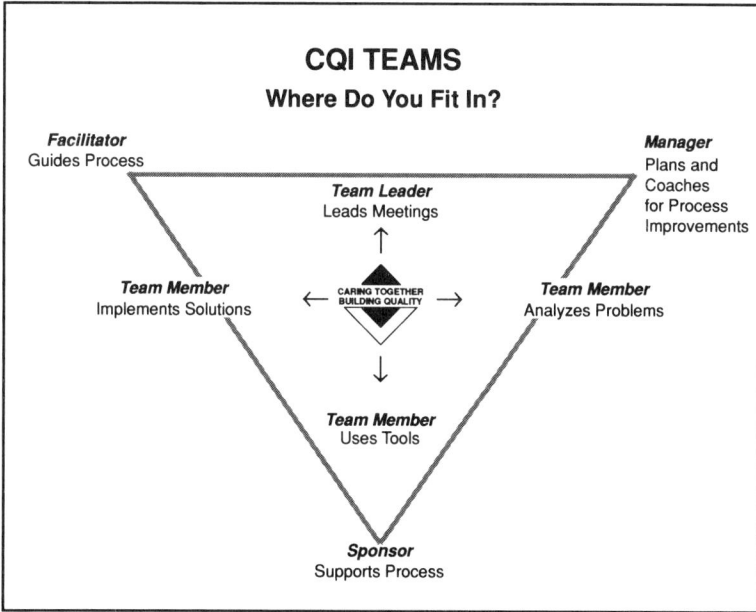

When teams are in their early stages of working together, it is not unusual to hear some misgivings expressed. "How do we know the physician just won't dominate everything? How many of us feel comfortable openly challenging a physician?" asked one participant. "What do medical records people have to do with treatment teams? I don't know if I could have anything to contribute there," said another. Some of the physicians raise questions about "bottom line" accountability. "Once an improvement idea is implemented, particularly if it deals directly with patients, who will be ultimately responsible if it doesn't work? In the public's eyes, if I am the physician in charge, *I* am the one held accountable," one physician observed.

Once teams gain the understanding that CQI projects do not subsume responsible medical decision-making or the obligations of health professionals' patient care roles, and that if there are things that go wrong, the data collected concerning the problem provide a reliable resource for finding out why, they are then able to focus their efforts on what becomes a win-win situation. They find better ways to facilitate each other's work and to continually improve service to patients and their families.

When teams learn the steps of the CQI pathway and are ready to begin a specific project, their immediate question is no doubt the same one the reader is by now asking: "Does it work?" As I observed earlier, total quality management cannot first be learned simply as a body of knowledge and then acted upon. Learning and doing are inextricably bound together. And so, just as important as the extensive CQI planning and educational programs at St. Joseph's was the simultaneous establishment of some initial demonstration projects.

DEMONSTRATION PROJECTS: FROM VISION TO ACTION
Translating total quality management from its visionary and philosophical basis to concrete implementation is without doubt the greatest challenge for any organization intent on placing itself on the total quality pathway. Needless to say, because total quality management moves hospitals in directions the implications of which no one can fully imagine, both internal hospital staff and external stakeholders such as government, community health organizations, and the general public, must become convinced that TQM is capable of delivering on its promises.

Around the time the education and training component of total quality management was launched, we also went through a process of choosing some specific CQI projects involving cross-functional teams. We saw these projects as active learning laboratories, demonstrating how the CQI methodology works in the team context.

Demonstration projects — and further CQI projects that come into being as total quality management begins to permeate the organization — allow the massive undertaking of implementing total quality management across the hospital to be broken down into manageable components. These projects not only result in some very real and effective changes, but also generate a good deal of excitement and enthusiasm among the teams and in the hospital as a whole.

St. Joseph's demonstration projects were the first hands-on experience of staff taking real ownership of improving the work processes in which they play a critical role. In my view, it is extremely important for hospitals in the early stages to choose these demonstration projects with care. They must be aimed at issues that have relevance to specific staff and to the organization as a whole. We call them "high pain" projects — that is, they are likely areas that staff and patients view as major barriers.

At the same time, they must not be projects so complex that evaluation is impossible. Nor should they be so massive in scope it would take years to see results. For example, the goal of a demonstration project should not be to totally reorganize the emergency department so that everything every day runs smoothly and efficiently and there are never any delays. Rather, the project should address specific aspects of emergency services, such as patient waiting time, ordering of tests, on-call staffing procedures, and so forth. In other words, the focus is on an improvement strategy that is "doable" and that, if successful, will make a significant difference to how work gets done.

The Quality Council at St. Joseph's has played a role in the selection of initial demonstration projects. We first reviewed existing information, including the Health Centre's strategic plan, its cross-functional annual goals and objectives, the results of patient satisfaction surveys, and the Canadian Council accreditation report for 1991-92.

We then used a method of brainstorming known as nominal group technique (NGT), by which a group of individuals "nominate" issues they feel deserve attention. The NGT method requires that members do not give each other comments or feedback during the initial listing of ideas. Preventing interaction at the early stage of idea collection ensures that participants will bring up issues that are of genuine concern to them. From an initial 46 suggestions, we chose three that we felt were particularly high pain for St. Joseph's and that we could improve using CQI.

Hospital parking, particularly difficulties getting into and out of the parking garage, was the target of some of the most common — and vocal — complaints from staff and patients alike. The chosen demonstration project was to come up with improvements in traffic flow.

The radiology department was the area chosen for another demonstration project. "Every hospital I know of complains about radiology — of patients having to wait for ages to get called down there or the slowness of getting the results back from procedures already done," observed George Labovitz at the October 1992 "Owning the Future" forum. Delays involving the radiology department at St. Joseph's were identified by the Quality Council as a major complaint area, leading to the establishment of a demonstration project aimed at finding ways to decrease the turn-around time of tests and the reporting of results.

The third demonstration project was to develop improved patterns of patient traffic in the operating rooms, the post-anaesthesia care unit, recovery room, and surgical day care. We saw this area as crucial to the delivery of future patient services at St. Joseph's, since much of the activity in these departments has implications for the high priority increasingly being placed upon ambulatory and outpatient care. After a time, a fourth demonstration project came into being to address another high pain aspect of hospital organization — patient waiting time in the emergency department.

The steps of continuous quality improvement — problem identification, flow charting, data gathering, and the identification and development of an improvement implementation plan — lend themselves well to the diagnostic model embedded within health care. The CQI teams assess problems or "symptoms" for their impact upon customers, and action is then taken to remedy these problems and improve the process overall. St. Joseph's demonstration projects are excellent illustrations of continuous quality improvement in action.

TEAMING UP TO TACKLE PROBLEMS

Each of the demonstration projects has followed its own time lines, data gathering, and evaluation strategies in developing plans for specific improvements. They report their key learnings and results on a quarterly basis to Quality Council and demonstrate a strong commitment to maintaining visibility throughout the Health Centre as a whole.

Patient Flow   The demonstration project involving patient flow in the operating rooms, post-anaesthesia care unit, and surgical day-care unit, was at first known at St. Joseph's as the OR/PACU/SDCU project. (This unwieldy acronym has been changed to simply the Surgical Team.) The team leader for the project is the PACU charge nurse. The facilitator is the supervisor of food services, and the project sponsor is the vice-president of patient services.

The process of getting patients from their hospital rooms to the operating rooms involves several hospital departments and many different staff. Initially, the team members were an operating room charge nurse, operating room staff nurse, post-anaesthetic care unit staff nurse, surgical day-care unit staff nurse, the manager of the surgical nursing unit, a surgeon, and an anaesthetist. Three months into the project, the team added a representative from portering and a surgical unit head nurse. The surgeon and anaesthetist continued their involvement on an ad hoc basis.

The team's first task was to create a flow chart of patients' movements from their hospital rooms to the operating rooms. The purpose was to uncover the reasons for delays in getting patients both to the operating room and from the operating room through PACU back to the nursing unit. From a patient (customer) perspective, delays in getting to the operating room often cause anxiety, uncertainty and annoyance. From a staff (internal customers) point of view, the delays are frustrating and often a factor in causing parts of the process to have to be repeated — for example, having to make a second telephone call from the OR area to the patient floor.

The team chose a variety of measurement tools — patient surveys, a survey of the surgeons and anaesthetists, and focus groups with nurses involved in the process.

"We found that patients themselves were not always the best gauge of how well we were doing in terms of timeliness to the OR," reflects team leader Jean Van Norden. "While many of them found the waiting to be an anxious time, they tended to push aside any frustrations with waiting in the light of just feeling relieved to get to the operating table itself, receive the right operation, and get it over with.

"It was from staff that we began to get information on delays. For example, we asked questions such as: Was it because the patient was in X-ray when the call from the OR came? Or perhaps it was because the telephone was busy on the floor and the call had to be repeated. Was it the lack of an available gurney to enable the porter to transport the patient to OR? The team decided to document primarily delays that were in excess of 15 minutes from the call to the unit to the departure of the patient to OR. As well, porters were asked to document delays of more than five minutes in travel time to the OR."

During a 19-day tracking period, the team found that while the majority of patients did reach the operating room within 20 minutes, there were significant numbers for whom the process took at least half an hour and some for whom the delay was more than 40 minutes. Similar findings were documented for the journey back from the OR to patients' rooms. "From there we determined our target levels of improvement for that aspect of the process: that the call to the unit until arrival at the OR should be accomplished within 20 minutes, and from the OR back to the room, a maximum time period of 15 minutes," explains Van Norden.

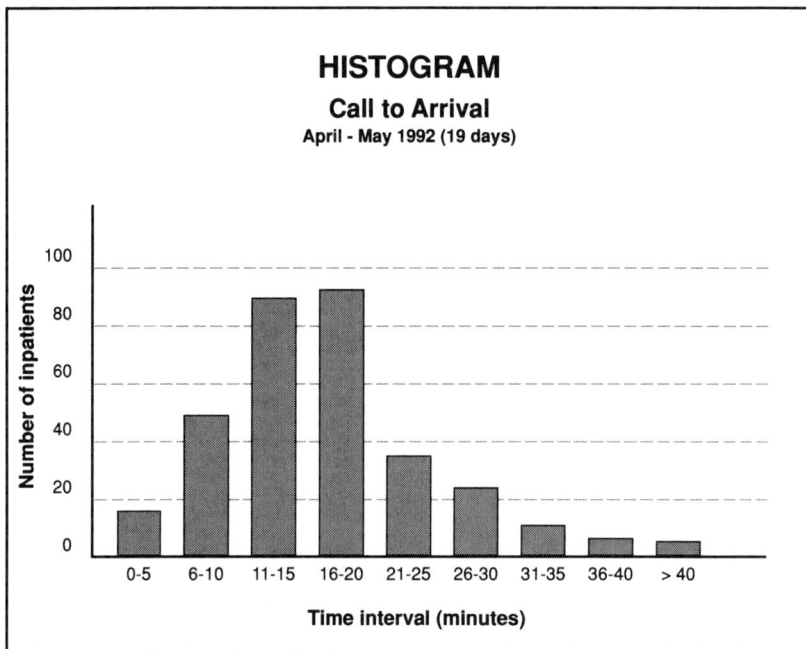

HISTOGRAM
Call to Arrival
April - May 1992 (19 days)

Number of inpatients

Time interval (minutes)

0-5 · 6-10 · 11-15 · 16-20 · 21-25 · 26-30 · 31-35 · 36-40 · > 40

    Van Norden and her team discovered enormous value in the cross-functional approach to improving quality. "When you can involve everyone who has a role in the process from its beginning to its end, it becomes far easier to work together to find solutions that work. The project has enabled us to better understand the customer focus of continuous quality improvement. By improving the timeliness of transporting patients, the patients benefit because they spend less anxious time just waiting and they feel their needs are being attended to. The staff, as internal customers, benefit from having the whole procedure run more smoothly. The OR teams have less problems with delays in scheduling, so that a more efficient operating room means less stress, streamlining the service for the OR team, and ultimately is more cost effective in that OR time is more efficiently used."

    Similarly, the emergency department demonstration project team was concerned with patient waiting time. With 45,000 patients seen annually in St. Joseph's emergency, a facility designed in the late 1950s to serve a maximum of 25,000 patients per year, it was not an unusual occurrence that the emergency department was often overcrowded and many patients were waiting several hours before being seen by medical staff.

Emergency Room   The emergency department project team looked at previous patient surveys concerning why patients leave the emergency area without being seen. They discovered that from patients' perspectives, there were three primary needs patients wanted satisfied: basic comfort such as food, warmth, security, and respect; clear communication about their care; and prompt service. The team also learned that patients expect to wait less than an hour to be seen by a physician and to be told of the reason for their wait if it is longer than this.

"We decided to focus on improving the quality of patient's waiting time," says team leader Jean Belbeck. "This is a very important point in that we didn't define the task as specifically 'cutting down' waiting times but more like, 'How do we ensure that our patients have a satisfactory experience of receiving service here?' Based on earlier evidence, improvements in the quality of the waiting time may well also accomplish reductions in patient waiting time. Improvements in the system just seem to grow naturally out of the total quality management customer focus."

The "earlier evidence" Belbeck refers to is that in 1990, emergency department staff began working with a new system they developed of fast tracking certain patients upon their arrival at the emergency department. Many of the long waits in hospital emergency departments involve patients with muscular or orthopedic injuries, such as ankle or wrist sprains, or broken bones. Physicians and emergency room staff at St. Joseph's collaborated to develop an expanded role for nurses who have been trained and certified to order such diagnostic tests as X-rays for common muscular and orthopedic injuries before the physician sees the patient. When the physician arrives, the X-ray results are already available and both patient and physician are not kept waiting for them.

"The patients feel that immediately upon their arrival, something is being done; someone is attending right away to their needs and concerns. The fast tracking has certainly increased the satisfaction levels of these patients," says Belbeck. "But another very positive benefit is that fast tracking has reduced patients' waiting time by an average of 40 minutes. From the average two-hour waiting time for patients with these types of injuries, the waiting period is now down to just over an hour and in many cases, it is between 30 and 60 minutes."

EMERGENCY ROOM STUDY
Time until Seen by Physician

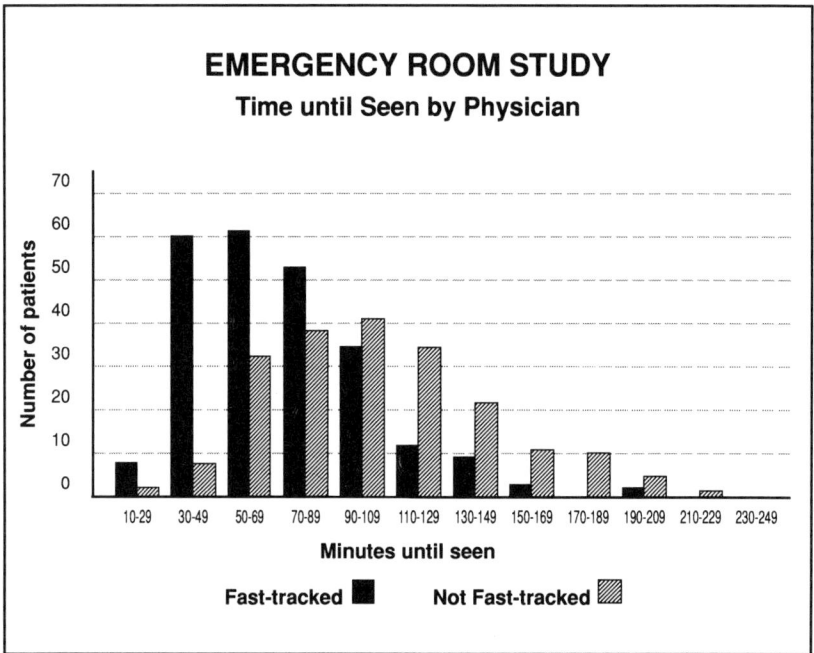

Building upon the success with the fast tracking of muscular and orthopedic injuries, the emergency department CQI team has identified opportunities for fast tracking other patients — for example, children with fevers, patients arriving to have their burns rechecked, or patients suffering allergy or asthma attacks. Further goals of the team include the development of a system for more clearly distinguishing urgent and nonurgent patients, and an improved communication system with patients — for example, a "reader friendly" brochure that explains to patients who gets seen first and what to expect.

The team also has a plan for the redesign of the emergency department itself, which will allow easier patient traffic flow and separate areas for urgent and nonurgent patients, with procedures in place for dealing with both. "Nothing is more frustrating than waiting to be seen in emergency and someone else gets in before you because their injury or illness is more serious than yours. Although you may understand why you have to wait, the situation just contributes to your anxiety. Every patient who comes to emergency feels his or her problem is urgent," says Belbeck. "Ultimately we want to have the most well-run, efficient, and effective emergency department possible. And success doesn't always lie only in the big changes. There are many things we can do for patients from the quality perspective — sometimes it is the small things, as well — something as simple as providing pillows, blankets, chairs, and magazines so that the waiting time is less stressful."

Radiology   The radiology demonstration project team also confronted a formidable challenge. This team chose its membership to include the special procedure technician, manager of radiology, senior transcriptionist, radiologist, radiology technician, clerk, film library clerk, and an orthopedic surgeon, as well as individuals filling the roles of facilitator, sponsor, and educator. Delays in the turnaround time for radiology patient reports is a constant frustration for many hospitals, and this was the initial focus of the radiology project team.

However, it soon became evident that the cause of many of the problems was not that radiology staff were inefficient; rather, the way the film library was organized created obstacles. In other words, the problem was in the process, not the people — a prime tenet of total quality management. The radiology project team readily reached a consensus that they could not effect a change in the turnaround time for reports without first solving the film library problem.

As its customers, the team identified all radiology staff, consultants and residents, nursing areas, outpatient departments, outside physicians, and other hospitals. The team defined three principal expectations of these customers. The first was that the location of radiological films be known.

"This issue was a real frustration in the department. There were gaps in how we tracked the films. Often they would be out in a department or with a physician, and the problem was that there were just too many places for the films to be," says radiology team leader Keith Butler. "If X-rays are 'lost' in this way, it can lead to tests being repeated — which is *not* good customer focus. Repeat tests cost the health system, as well as expose patients unnecessarily to radiation."

The second customer expectation was the need for radiological reports to be processed as soon as possible after a test is done. The third expectation was that there be a better system to ensure accessibility of radiological films and reports. Over a three-week period in February

1992, the team tracked problems encountered on radiology requisition forms and recorded these on a bar graph. By far the most frequent problem was that a good number — almost 200 requisitions — did not indicate the ordering physician's name. Lesser problems, ones that nevertheless affected up to 50 requisitions during the period, included the wrong spelling of the patient's name, missing health card numbers, missing birth date and address.

The team created a second bar graph illustrating the results of tracking the location of radiological films during a one-week period. Thirty-three were found in the emergency department, with the next greatest numbers being located in the hand and upper-limb outpatient centre (29), and in doctors' offices (23). Often these films had been there for some time and had not been returned to the radiology department.

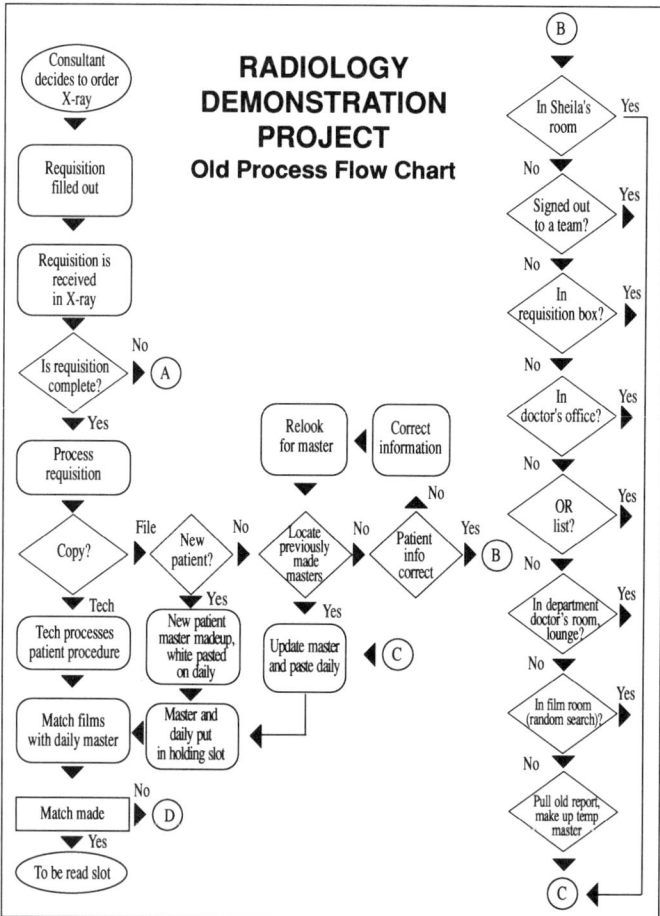

RADIOLOGY DEMONSTRATION PROJECT
Old Process Flow Chart

After making an elaborate flow chart of the radiology film process beginning from the physician's order for an X-ray, the team then charted the film library process involving scheduled patients and another chart for the request for films. Team members then designed a new process flow chart they believed would work better.

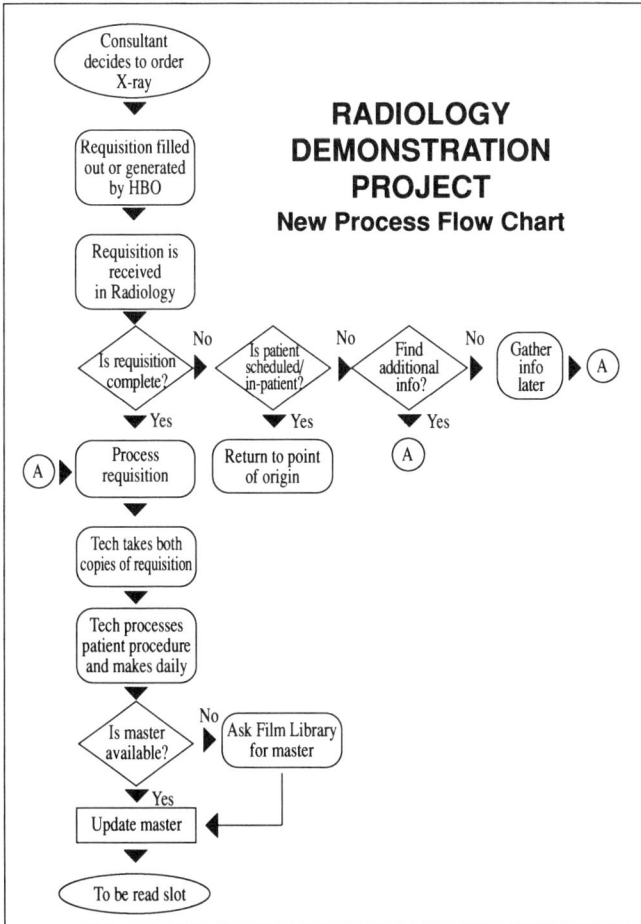

RADIOLOGY DEMONSTRATION PROJECT
New Process Flow Chart

Using the new process flow chart as a sort of map, the team began implementation of their improvement plan. Clearly written film-request forms and the close involvement of a booking clerk in the requisition process became a central strategy. The existing filing systems were reduced from three to one. The team instituted a daily list to track unreported films and made individual doctors' slots. For scheduled patients, films were pulled the night before. There is now also a sign-out system for X-ray masters and a stamp to identify films if they are leaving the department, a process change that should make tracking the unreported films easier.

The next phase of the radiology project has involved gathering data on the results of the process changes in the film library and further refining the improvements. "We learned that this type of improvement process takes time and patience," says Butler. "But it is more than worth it when staff who work at individual aspects of the process realize that, working together, we are capable of creating real improvements that will make a difference in how we serve the Health Centre's patients and staff."

Hospital Parking   The parking garage improvement team concentrated its initial efforts on dealing with peak arrival times of staff. Some staff members were asked to consider altering their start time by 15 minutes as one way of alleviating parking garage congestion in the mornings. The team also asked the City of London to move the taxi stands on the parking garage street. This, too, has reduced congestion. A new automated card reader has been installed in the garage that accurately tracks the number of vehicles in the garage at any time. For the longer term, the parking garage team is evaluating two alternative plans for building a new parking garage entrance.

Some of the demonstration projects were overdesigned. That was in part to learn from them. Some, it may be suggested, have taken too long to improve processes. These are some of the things learned from this approach.

THE TOTAL QUALITY MANAGEMENT INFLUENCE
BEGINS TO SPREAD

As more and more staff members became familiar with, and trained in, continuous quality improvement tools and methods, we began to see the outgrowth of that process in the creation of new continuous quality improvement teams. The experience of success with specific CQI projects, and the communication of those successes throughout the hospital, began rapidly to boost morale and create enthusiasm for change. Staff perceive, as Keith Butler says, that it is possible to make a difference, or as Jean Belbeck has observed, that often major successes are achieved through seemingly small or simple changes.

Further improvement projects have been established in many ways and in many areas of St. Joseph's, and there will no doubt be numerous others as organizational culture shifts to total quality management. Sometimes staff have gained confidence first with departmental improvement projects. In the pharmacy department, for example, front-line staff felt they needed more than the eight-hour "Your Role in Quality" training. The training was expanded to a ninth session so that staff and management could review key learnings and address issues specific to the planning projects for the pharmacy department. With this increased confidence, the department initiated about 20 of its own small "mini-demonstration" projects.

"The projects had to be small enough to achieve change within three months and wide enough in scope for us to see that they make a difference overall," says Director of Pharmacy Chris Judd who has played a key role in the CQI training of pharmacy staff.

Among the small, but nonetheless important, achievements in the pharmacy department's CQI initiatives has been the creation of an improved method for keeping minutes of meetings, a revised system for recording telephone messages, and the elimination of the waste resulting from paper bags used to transport drugs to hospital floors and their replacement with reusable insulated bags.

"I like to compare the learning of continuous quality improvement methods to learning to drive," says Judd. "When you're new at the wheel, you practise on empty parking lots and side streets. Then you go for the busier main roads."

The comfort level achieved with the small projects has allowed for several larger departmental pharmacy improvement projects, among them a team looking at the issue of space for the department, another dealing with how the role of pharmacy is viewed at the hospital, and a team whose goal is to create a consistent standardization of the procedures by which pharmacy deals with other hospital departments.

Pharmacy also became closely involved with several of the cross-functional CQI teams at St. Joseph's. Experiences similar to that of the pharmacy department are becoming increasingly evident throughout the Health Centre. From small departmental projects to cross-functional clinical teams to corporate improvement projects, a creative synergy and sense of excitement and challenges have been built up, which fuel the impetus to develop further improvement projects. Total quality management creates energy in an organization, and change comes to be seen more as an opportunity for improvement and innovation than as a reason for stress and uncertainty.

There are now 15 major cross-functional teams formally established at

St. Joseph's, with more coming on board each week. The initial four demonstration projects are nearing completion. The newer continuous quality improvement projects involve both clinical services and support services. There are numerous other small projects (but we no longer keep track of small projects because they're so numerous) aimed at improving processes, and staff are justifiably proud of the results.

The operating room/central processing team, for example, is working to eliminate unnecessary steps in the cleaning and sterilization of operating room instruments and there is a team to co-ordinate the policies and processes involving service uniforms. A food-and-nutrition servery team is evaluating the future role of food serveries throughout St. Joseph's.

On the clinical side, the episiotomy team has as its key goal the elimination of unnecessary episiotomies. A dialysis team is streamlining the treatment protocols of the dialysis process.

One particularly major organizational challenge for hospitals is the process of discharge planning. "At St. Joseph's we came to realize that improvements to discharge planning could not be one huge CQI project. The area is so complex that it has been divided into three projects — medical/surgical discharge planning, complex-cases discharge planning, and early-response discharge planning," says Chris Judd, the pharmacy representative on the discharge planning improvement teams.

Effective discharge planning is crucial to a hospital's efficiency and quality of care. The benefits to a hospital of technological advances, such as laparoscopic surgery, and clinical care improvements, which have succeeded in accomplishing a much shorter length of stay for many patients, can be impeded by less than efficient medical/surgical discharge planning.

Imagine for a moment that you are a patient who has had heart surgery. The medical team has determined that you have recovered enough to be discharged from hospital, and you cannot wait to get home. But there is a delay of some hours in getting the discharge order written. Perhaps the order is written in late morning and it will be at least 6 p.m. before you can leave. The result? You end up occupying a hospital bed almost a day longer than necessary. Again, the problem lies not in people — everyone is doing what they are supposed to be doing, that is, getting the paperwork ready, calling your family to arrange for your transportation home, and so forth — but the problem is in the process, the system by which patient discharge is organized.

St. Joseph's medical/surgical discharge team has defined as its central goal the shortening of the gap between the expected time of discharge and the actual time of discharge. "We have to analyse what the blocks to efficient discharge are and then modify the system to eliminate them. It could be something as simple as having all discharge orders written the night before instead of keeping the patient waiting just for the paper to be signed the next day," says Judd. "It could be notifying family or making transportation arrangements the day before discharge, so that these support systems are ready when the patient is."

The discharge of complex-care patients constitutes an even greater challenge for hospitals. When a patient's condition is very complex — for example, when he or she has suffered serious complications from a disease, has had an adverse reaction to a medical procedure, or has an illness/condition that will require continuing care out in the community — the discharge planning process takes much more time. Many complex cases involve the frail elderly whose discharge is burdened by the necessity of finding them placement in adequate community care facilities.

Many physicians, nursing staff, and hospital administrators know the frustration of having patients fill acute-care hospital beds while waiting for an opening in a community facility. While I do not mean to imply that the improvement of an individual hospital's discharge process with these patients will totally solve the larger health care system problem of the availability of chronic- and long-term-care beds or of in-home community care programs, an effective process in acute-care hospitals for the timely, safe, and efficient discharge of complex-care patients will be a significant help in reducing pressure on the system as a whole.

"The relationship to quality improvement overall, I think, is that we are looking to identify these patients well ahead of time and institute the discharge planning process very early on," says Judd. "My role, for example, has to do with the management of patients' drugs. From a pharmacy perspective, a patient is deemed a complex case when he or she is on six or more medications. Pharmacy has to become involved early on; we have to know their admitting diagnosis, what has happened during hospitalization, and potential drug interactions and toxicities."

The other discharge planning project at St. Joseph's, the early-response discharge planning team, is gathering data on the process for dealing with elderly patients who arrive at the hospital's emergency department with a health crisis but for whom admission to hospital is not the most appropriate measure. The team's goal is to make improvements to the system that will result in a satisfactory solution for these patients.

This whole discharge planning process review, which is very complex and extremely important to the hospitals of the future, will eventually lead to the system's review of care from admission of the patient (or even earlier) to care back in the community, with an eye on ways to improve the process.

THE NEED TO EXTEND CQI INTO THE COMMUNITY

As continuous quality improvement projects, particularly those that focus on patient care, become more numerous at St. Joseph's, the need to move CQI's concepts further into the community has become evident. St. Joseph's is currently playing a key role in creating one such comprehensive hospital/community CQI project. In collaboration with a major Canadian pharmaceutical company, St. Joseph's is developing a "self-administration of medication" (SAM) initiative, involving the hospital, community health agencies, and community pharmacies.

At the hospital, the project focuses on the development of clearer, more consistent teaching of patients concerning the drugs prescribed for them. Those patients identified as good candidates for SAM — those who appear most receptive to participating in a shared decision-making approach to health care — will, while still in hospital, be taught to self-administer their medications with appropriate coaching from hospital staff.

In the community, the project is creating a support system that will be effective in dealing with medication difficulties very quickly. This may take the form of a 24-hour hot-line which patients can call for immediate assistance if they become concerned about dosage levels, their reaction to a drug, or any other issue concerning their medications. But the most unique aspect of the project is the involvement of community pharmacists.

The usual procedure for a pharmacist when confronted by a customer raising a concern about a drug's side-effects is to instruct the customer to get in touch with his or her doctor. The aim of the self-administered medication project is that a pharmacist will call the hotline and then immediately pass specific instructions on to the customer. Since approximately two to fifteen per cent of readmissions to hospital are due to adverse drug reactions, particularly among the elderly, there is much to be gained from being able to deal with patients' medication concerns on the spot, rather than waiting until the situation becomes a crisis requiring admission to hospital through the emergency department.

While there have been programs such as medication hotlines — for example, in Manitoba — and research done on drug reactions among the elderly, I believe the self-administered medication project jointly run by St. Joseph's, the pharmaceutical industry, and the community is one of the first Canadian programs to approach the prescription of drugs, patients' shared decision-making in taking the drugs, and the community's role in providing information resources in a comprehensive, customer-focused manner.

"There is enormous potential for putting the data-gathering tools of continuous quality improvement to work in the community," claims Linda Kulkarni, St. Joseph's senior consultant for nursing research. "Hospital/community collaboration in the care of patients is currently a strong priority in public policy. As we have moved to much shorter lengths of stay in hospital and more emphasis on home care, now more than ever we need good evaluation tools to give us accurate information on what is most effective for patients and on what enables community health agencies to serve patients in terms of quality of care and customer satisfaction."

CQI tools and strategies are being used in current nursing research at St. Joseph's, evaluating from a community perspective the process of patients making the transition from hospital to home. These include analyses of trends such as readmission rates within three months, and of the obstacles to the effectiveness and efficiency of the interagency network required to deliver high-quality community health services to patients.

Very often, policy changes regarding community care and hospital/community co-ordination are driven by the provincial ministries of health, which are motivated more by questions of cost effectiveness rather than by what communities actually need, or even more importantly, by what will work in specific communities. Because quality improvement measurement and analysis methods can be quite readily learned by the individuals, groups, and organizations whose responsibility it is to administer and deliver health care in communities, in future, we should be able to use quality improvement strategies to achieve significant, positive changes in the policy-making arena of health care. Total quality management can eventually permeate not just our hospitals, but all health care agencies and health care funding bodies, and we can begin to create a health care system that delivers a seamless, continually improving, high quality of care from the community to the hospital and back into the community.

6

Maintaining the Impact of Total Quality Management

The CQI message is so seductive because it is so obvious and so simple. The reality is very different; confronting and hard. The results can be staggering for those with the consistency of purpose, the courage and determination to follow it through fully. The fact that something is simple does not mean it is easy.

— MIKE ROBSON, MANAGING DIRECTOR,
MRA INTERNATIONAL

Labour relations, reward and recognition, communications, and long-term evaluation are as much part of St. Joseph's Health Centre's total quality management story as the work of our continuous quality improvement teams in all areas of the hospital. Together, they create the impetus and motivation for change. The adage "the whole is greater than the sum of the parts" is never more true than in the achievement of a culture of total quality management within health institutions.

If TQM is to work, hospital labour relations must be brought into alignment with our commitment to quality. The strike at the CAMI automotive plant in fall 1992 illustrates just how formidable a task this is. According to many of the media reports on that strike, it was evident that management and union had very different definitions of the term "participative management" and that prior to the strike, union-management interactions at CAMI, which had been viewed as a Canadian model of Japanese management methods, had become increasingly confrontational and adversarial. Labour relations is, without doubt, one of the severest testing grounds for total quality management.

Another area is the issue of reward and recognition of staff. Organizational experts today repeatedly warn that the days of employee subservience and deference to authority are long gone; as Peter Drucker says in his article "The New Society of Organizations," "Loyalty can no longer be obtained by the paycheck." In particular, it is foolish for hospitals to assume that health care workers will feel sufficiently recognized by pleasant-sounding words about the value of health care in society and their role in the system given the great stress placed upon the health care delivery by increased demands and resource restraints.

A third area the success of total quality management depends upon is communications. Good communication strategies, which are highly valued by many businesses and industries today, are absolutely crucial to such public institutions as hospitals, in the throes of making significant changes in the context of the current social climate of economic turmoil and public cynicism.

Lastly, and perhaps most importantly, is the area of evaluation. If hospitals become committed to total quality management as the way of the future and take steps to implement these changes, there needs to be in place a system for evaluating outcomes. "How will we know it's really working and making a difference?" and "How long until we see results in terms of better-run programs or significant cost savings?" are questions frequently asked by continuous quality improvement teams. Hospitals, and the health care system itself, will lose the momentum for change in the direction of total quality management unless a process of continuous evaluation, which provides answers to these questions, is a crucial part of the TQM initiative.

Union-Management Relations Of St. Joseph's Health Centre's 3,200 employees, 1,800 are unionized, and there are nine bargaining units in total. Union representatives have been part of developing the vision of total quality management since early in the process.

The commitment to positive union-management relations at St. Joseph's predates the total quality management initiative. We have a long tradition of acknowledging the value and dignity of all our staff, though in the past couple of decades the Health Centre has had its share of labour turmoil. This turmoil is reflective of the growing uneasiness and conflict in the economic and workplace climate and of the rapidly developing changes in the direction of the health care system. In 1986, however, we successfully achieved a settlement with our bargaining units when many other hospitals at that time had gone to arbitration. This event, says St. Joseph's director of personnel Paul Faguy, helped reinforce a growing trend toward more open union-management communications.

My strong interest in and experience with quality of work life at Foothills Hospital continued upon my arrival at St. Joseph's. This became more formalized, or designed into, the Health Centre's organizational culture through an emphasis on establishing a Quality of Work Life Steering Committee at St. Joseph's in 1989.

The Quality of Work Life Steering Committee today is a model of the collaborative and cross-functional mix that characterizes total quality management. From patient services come five employees and one union executive member; from technical/allied health are three employees and one union executive member; from the service department, three employees and one union executive member; one representative from clerical; two representatives from senior administration, the Director of Personnel and the Director of Total Quality Management; and one secretary from the administrative area.

It encompasses many areas of staff experience at St. Joseph's, including organizing employees' charitable contributions, playing a role in long-term service recognition awards, the development of a child care program, the creation of an employee handbook that includes a TQM perspective, staff development fund, a discount booklet offering price discounts at several local businesses, and an ongoing "new ideas" initiative.

The positive gains for St. Joseph's staff accomplished by the Quality of Work Life Steering Committee have helped to build bridges toward the union-management relationship envisioned in total quality management. The phrases "union-management partnering" or "union-management collaboration" are often met with employee cynicism in the current economic and business climate of "lean and mean" bottom-line competitiveness. As early as 1989, we recognized that if we really wanted to change the culture to be more open and collaborative, the traditional concepts of labour relations would have to be challenged and significantly altered.

At many workplaces, both in the public and private sectors, the union-management model is trapped in the bureaucratic hierarchies of the past. Faguy calls this model one in which "Management acts — Union reacts."

At the October 1992 "Owning the Future" conference in Toronto, he described the traditional roles of management as "plan, organize, direct, control, co-ordinate." The traditional roles of unions, he says, are first to improve working conditions, second to protect gains already accomplished such as salary levels or job security, and third to influence the employer in decision-making — how work is organized and how it is recompensed.

In Chapter Three, I talked about the us versus them mentality that frequently characterizes physician-administration relations in hospitals. But the us versus them mind-set is even more widespread between unions and administration; and TQM leaders must address it. Typical of this mind-set is the management view that unions and their concerns get in the way of allowing them to run the business or institution smoothly, and the union view that management does not really care about them, only about how they can get more for less money.

Sheldon Bumstead, a medical technologist in hematology and immunohematology, chairman of one of St. Joseph's union chapters, and chairman of the Quality of Work Life Steering Committee, was a workshop leader on union-management partnership at the Toronto conference. He described the need to move from a model of confrontation to one of collaboration if total quality management is to work. Pointing out that one of the dictionary definitions of the word "collaboration" is "working with the enemy," he emphasized in the workshop that collaboration does not always mean agreeing, but rather, seeks the achievement of concrete positive outcomes for both sides through good-faith negotiations and workable compromises.

Both management and unions experience significant ambivalence and fear around such issues as potential loss of control and possible hidden agendas. For example, a manager may give lip service to the concept of union-management partnership but really intend only to return to business as usual. Or a union representative may take a certain position on an issue because he or she is concerned with re-election to a union office. Some union members are uneasy about the marriage of union and management that appears to take place in total quality management. Both management and union representatives may feel they go through participative discussions often with no clearly defined outcome.

TQM postulates an entirely different management-employee model. Increasingly in the 1990s and beyond, organizational experts say, good management will entail the ability of working both with and through individuals to accomplish common goals. Total quality management is an acknowledgement of the value of everyone's role within the organization and represents an evolution from win-lose labour negotiations to win-win.

Total quality management does not view labour relations from the short-term perspective but chooses, rather, the view of the longer term. It aligns its labour negotiations approach with its future vision of excellence and the achievement of total quality. It will not work if labour relations are acrimonious. This is not to say that in the new paradigm of TQM, there are never any disputes, but that the communications strategy is one of good faith, openness, and honesty in the search for equitable solutions to problems of concern to unions, management, and the hospital as a whole.

What's in it for Union Leaders? The greatest tool total quality management has to offer labour relations is subtle but dramatic in its influence — the focus on processes that lead to measurable outcomes. In other words, in a negotiating process, neither management nor unions concentrate on the number of disagreements or conflicts concerning specific issues, but instead on whether or not the negotiations can be successful in achieving a satisfactory outcome for all parties. Of course, in the current climate of funding restraints and downsizing, this is not to say that the solutions can be perfect.

Since 1986, there has been a steady trend toward contract negotiations at St. Joseph's being settled by agreement rather than arbitration. In 1992, 100 per cent of contract negotiations concluded with agreements. At a two-day seminar held at the Health Centre in November 1992 on total quality management in health care, attended by representatives of approximately 15 Ontario hospitals and other health care agencies, one participant asked union representative John McDonald if the reason for this was a reflection of generalized societal anxiety about job security, the mind-set that says, "Hold onto this job because you might not get another one."

"*No*," responded McDonald emphatically. "There were other hospitals going to arbitration despite the job climate. The settlements were because we believed that together we had arrived at an arrangement that would work for everyone."

TRENDS IN NEGOTIATIONS

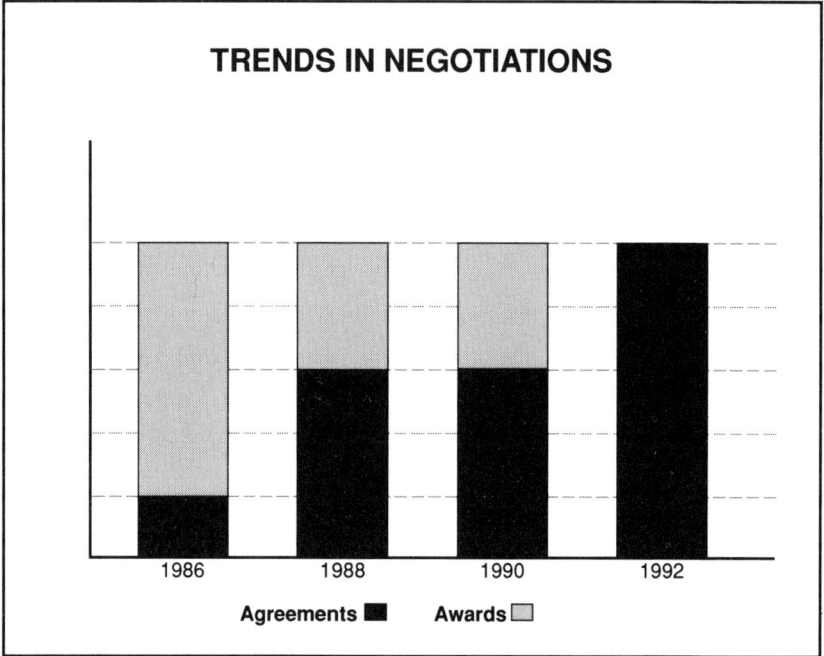

1986   1988   1990   1992

Agreements ■   Awards ▨

TRENDS IN GRIEVANCE ACTIVITY

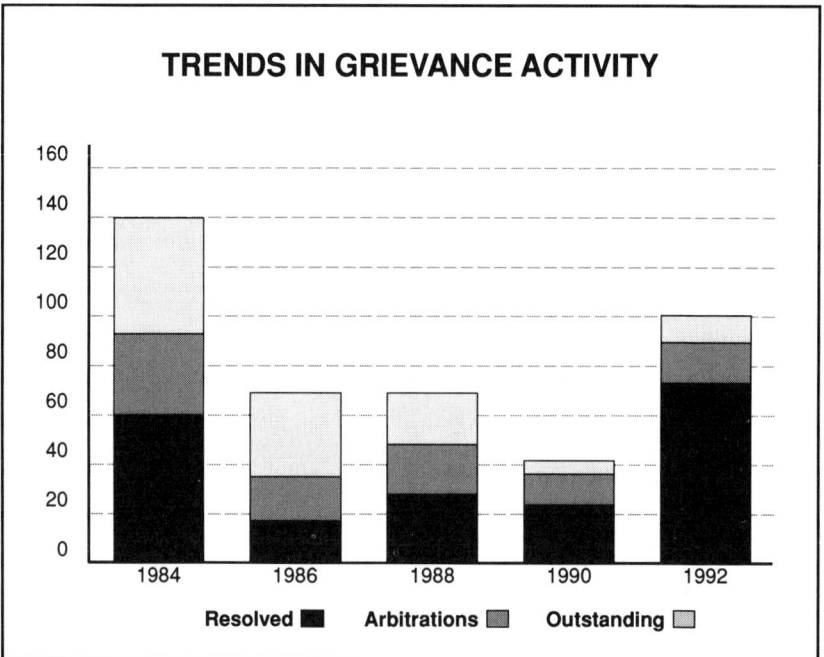

1984   1986   1988   1990   1992

Resolved ■   Arbitrations ▨   Outstanding ▨

There is also a results-oriented trend evident in the handling of grievances. Of approximately 100 grievance situations in 1992, more than 80 were resolved without arbitration, as opposed to 1984, when of 140 grievances, less than half were resolved without arbitration. Between 1990 and 1992, grievance situations went up somewhat — most likely reflecting in part the "crazy time" turmoil connected with the introduction of TQM as the new organizational direction — but a far greater percentage of grievances in 1992 were resolved without arbitration than was the case in 1990.

It has become the practice at St. Joseph's that union representatives, along with board members, physicians, department managers, and senior management, participate in strategic planning meetings. As well, periodic information sessions are held for all staff to discuss the current operating plan and the financial realities at the Health Centre for the coming year.

Trust and openness in the thorny and often controversial field of labour relations cannot be accomplished overnight, nor can the win-win mentality take hold instantly. But an honest commitment to total quality management on both sides has placed St. Joseph's on a new level of collaboration among all staff groups, a state of affairs that bodes well for the hospital's ability to respond proactively and in the interests of all its internal stakeholders. It has resulted in members of management and the nine bargaining units to gain a clearer and more positive understanding of their roles. Total quality management has, as Senge puts it, "given us a place to go," a new collaborative vision to strive for in the area of hospital labour relations.

But because this whole process, this way of thinking, is relatively new, there are situations where one failure in trust will cause dissolution of the partnership. Thus, talking to each union person when there are rumours or misunderstandings, is vital. If we are to contribute to the health of our society, we need to mature our working relationships. I have been as disappointed in some senior managers and their backroom sniping at unions as I have been with union leaders who are unable to give managers an opportunity or room to improve their relationship with unions. This is a very tough situation to reverse. But with a measure of integrity, trust and will to do so, mature people are capable of becoming visionary and solution-focused, and thus can discard the fears and worries of unhelpful, if not destructive, relationships. If we dig deep enough into each other's perceptions, we do share many similar goals.

Communication and the commitment to a consistent purpose by all is

an absolute necessity to make a collaborative union-management partnership work. Mike Mullin, president of the local Ontario Nurses Association
at St. Joseph's Health Centre, has been extremely effective at consciously
raising issues needing dialogue. He has walked into my office, never
inappropriately, whenever the organization's tempo or stress level required clarification or when an issue needed more attention. He has
worked extremely well with managers, vice-presidents, directors of nursing, and personnel to achieve a better workplace for his members. Yet he
always makes clear his union's position on issues.

He and the leaders from other unions have my trust, and they are a
large part of what makes St. Joseph's such a good place to work. Our
recent acknowledgement in London Business Monthly Magazine as one
of the top ten London workplaces (and the largest employer of the top
ten) testifies to how far we have come in creating collaborative union-
management relationships.

REWARD AND RECOGNITION

The Canadian public has high expectations of health care professionals.
So, too, do the organizations in which these professionals work. The
challenges of delivering high-quality health care in an increasingly demanding and complex environment fall directly onto health care providers. As well, those who are responsible for the wide variety of support
services within health institutions, such as dietary, clerical, housekeeping,
and maintenance must also perform excellent work so that the work of
those who directly care for patients can be properly accomplished. In
many cases, these individuals are taken even more for granted because
much of their work is invisible. Patients tend to assume that such services
are in place and running well, but don't give a thought to why that is so.

Total quality management in health care institutions places further
expectations upon everyone — administration, care providers, and support staff — to take direct ownership of the processes aimed at the
continuous improvement of services. Total quality management cannot
work without the commitment, time, and talents of people; and in health
care, these people are extremely busy and often very pressured. As a
philosophy and practice that is value-driven, TQM includes systems that
recognize and reward the dedication and contributions of staff who, in the
pursuit of excellence and total quality in everything they do, often go the
extra mile for their patients and for each other. Also implicit in TQM is

that individuals and teams must be recognized for consistent good work that moves the institution incrementally further and further along the road to total quality.

The Quality Climate Survey conducted at St. Joseph's Health Centre in 1991 identified reward and recognition of staff as a key area in need of improvement. Almost 40 per cent of survey respondents disagreed with the statement "My management provides praise when I do high quality work." In terms of teamwork, 41 per cent disagreed that management recognizes and rewards groups or teams who perform high-quality work. And on both questions, a significant percentage — almost 20 per cent — chose to remain neutral, neither agreeing nor disagreeing.

In response to these concerns, a task force on reward and recognition was formed in April 1992. Grounding its purpose within TQM values, the task force adopted as its goal a 20 per cent improvement of positive staff perceptions of reward and recognition by the next Quality Climate Survey in 1993.

Over 100 members of Health Centre staff participated in a series of focus groups to define what the concepts "recognition" and "reward" meant to them. They described recognition generally as the acknowledgement of their efforts and contributions, the giving of praise and respect, positive and constructive criticism, and appreciation for their daily work. One staff member defined it as simply "someone appreciates you and lets you know it."

Reward, on the other hand, was seen as a process of formal recognition such as days off, receiving an award, education leave, and financial incentives. "Reward is a tangible thing — it should be measurable," said one staff member. Many thought it should be written commendations included in personnel files, a public announcement, or bulletin display. Others felt it should include "perks, incentives, and bonuses similar to industry." For many focus group participants, reward and recognition were closely linked, as in the comment of one person, "Recognition is the starting point for reward; recognition and reward go hand in hand."

Two main themes emerged from the focus groups. Staff wanted recognition both for consistent good work — which has always been expected of health care staff — and for their excellence, innovation, and demonstrated commitment to TQM, including their ability to lead successfully amidst change and adapt to or create new ideas.

The focus group participants identified already existing successful reward and recognition programs at St. Joseph's Health Centre such as the Sisters of St. Joseph Award, given for consistent excellence in care and compassion; Long-Term Service Awards; staff development and education funds; retirement teas; and thank-you letters.

The task force, acting on the results of the focus groups felt that many of the current programs could be expanded. In addition, staff were given some specific education on how to give and receive recognition.

The expansion of reward and recognition at St. Joseph's Health Centre to reflect a TQM focus includes both short-term and long-term strategies. Short-term are actions that are immediate and often spontaneous — for example, the creation of "I noticed" cards in which a staff member acknowledges something a colleague did that was admired and respected, or hand-written thank-you cards from one department to another or one individual to another. St. Joseph's pharmacy department, for example, has developed a recognition "chain letter," in which one staff member communicates appreciation to another staff member; the recipient then looks for an opportunity to pass the letter on to another colleague, and so forth.

The task force has also looked at creating "thank-you grams," by which a fellow employee, supervisor, visitor, or patient sends a note of appreciation and a duplicate copy to the staff member's immediate supervisor or a Staff Recognition Task Force.

Some of the long-term reward and recognition strategies being adopted by St. Joseph's Health Centre take the form of highly noticeable poster boards recognizing entire departments, offering coaching-skills development opportunities through educational services, an annual-staff-appreciation day for every department, and the recognition through group photos of departments achieving outstanding customer service.

Other long-term plans ensure that reward and recognition is grounded in the values and practices of total quality management and focuses especially on team performance as well as individuals. All employee suggestions for improvement, for example, receive written acknowledgement and feedback from the Quality of Work Life Steering Committee. A recognition system has been developed to acknowledge contributions or innovations in quality, patient care, the enhancement of the quality of work life, and cost-savings. Several of the task force's recommendations include rewarding and recognizing innovations by individuals or teams that result in cost-savings. One initiative is that a percentage of realized savings may be given to the employee or the department. Another is the potential for hospital-wide gain-sharing based on the achievement of cost reductions beyond required targets.

While we cannot provide monetary rewards directly to unionized staff because of contracts, we must create ways of exceeding their expectations. In both 1990 and 1991 we exceeded our annual objectives. Clearly the staff needed to be rewarded. As a result we provided $50,000 to the Quality of Work Life Steering Committee to use for creating development opportunities they saw as important for the people working at St. Joseph's. The manner in which the members of the committee managed the fund made me extremely proud of their competence and reinforced my confidence in them.

This idea was enthusiastically adopted by the Board. The QWL Committee members have been judicious and thoughtful concerning how they use the funds. Under present union contracts, we cannot reward staff in the same way. We plan to provide the $50,000 each year to the QWL committee when financial and other major goals are met, in recognition that management cannot achieve effective results in the organization without every employee's efforts.

At the same time, two per cent of every manager's potential income is made available and provided to *all* or *none* of them at the end of the year depending upon whether we meet the goals of the big team, that is, all of management's key objectives. This is an amount not large enough to cause negative feelings about team results, yet positive enough to encourage the teams to achieve results.

In summary, the Reward and Recognition Task Force drew from St. Joseph's mission statement that states in part, "we foster a work environment that values the contribution of each person." Our recognition and reward system focuses on moving both our objectives and organizational values forward. Our primary emphasis continues to be on *recognition* rather than monetary rewards, and on team accomplishments as well as individual accomplishments.

Six principles guide St. Joseph's recognition and reward system:

- appreciation
- contribution
- genuineness
- participation
- simplicity
- celebration

These principles affirm the creativity and commitment of individuals and groups in the continuous pursuit of improvements in service and organizational processes. The phrase "People are your greatest asset" is heard often in business and industry, and other public institutions, particularly those who recognize the need to attract and hold highly competent "knowledge workers."

EVALUATING PERFORMANCE DIFFERENTLY

One of our most important reward and recognition efforts has been to redesign the performance appraisal system. While this has yet to be fully accomplished, senior managers have started to realign the performance improvement reviews to focus more on key customers and outcomes. The person to whom the vice-presidents report reviews their performance, but colleagues and subordinates also provide constructive improvement ideas as part of the review.

This is an extremely vital new direction. It reinforces the idea that people are not the problem but that systems are. And it emphasizes that we can continually improve what we do in the eyes of those we serve. All of the vice-presidents now assess their performance in this way — as I do. It is fair to say that of all the people who know best how the vice-presidents are functioning, I am usually the last to know. Therefore, the best way for the vice-presidents to improve their performance is to be given honest, specific feedback from colleagues and subordinates, and to address those things which cannot be easily talked about except in a safe zone, or which might be deemed to be off the record.

But the commitment to recognize and reward people for their contributions to a better workplace and a better future must not remain in the realm of talk. It must be translated to action.

Communications   Without attention given to the central role of communications, quality improvement strategies will rapidly lose their impact, particularly in organizations as complex as hospitals. The strategies must be communicated in the hospital in ways that reinforce perceptions that TQM is the established approach to service delivery among staff, physicians, volunteers, and their customers, internal and external.

What is a learning opportunity if it is not a powerful form of communication? Communication is so intrinsic to the implementation of TQM that it is hard to separate implementation from communication. Educating staff, building teams, developing a vision, and recognizing achievements are initiatives that succeed only with effective dialogue and the sharing of important information.

Communication in an organization committed to total quality management is a long-term process and must constantly be scrutinized for its effect. There always needs to be an impetus to both maintain and reinforce TQM values throughout the organization. At St. Joseph's, one of our earliest steps was to develop a strategic communications plan. What we strive to communicate are the values and practices of the total quality management process. We are not just filling the function of transmitting information; we are going further than that. Motivating staff to think and act with total quality management in mind requires a new and wider understanding of the role of communications.

It is common for many hospitals these days to have public relations departments and such communications vehicles as newsletters, brochures, magazines, photographic displays, and bulletin boards, as well as press releases sent to external media. Within the framework of total quality management, however, these tools need to be reframed and incorporated into a more broad-ranging communications strategy that will define and enrich the vision of the organization. This vision directs itself to both internal and external audiences.

Imagine communications as a solid platform upon which rest the values and vision of total quality management. From this platform, every issue, large or small, is communicated in the context of the whole — not only of the hospital but of the community at large. Every communications activity — from a simple conversation that imparts some needed information to the glossiest of hospital magazines or annual reports to the colourful images of a well-produced video — will paint a compelling verbal and visual picture of the Health Centre as it aligns and integrates each one of its departments and patient care programs with total quality management.

Effective communications succeed not only in informing people about changes or certain specific issues, but also help each member of the organization gain an appreciation for the Health Centre staff's ongoing direct role in managing change and delivering high quality care to the community.

At St. Joseph's we reviewed our existing communications strategies in order to identify opportunities for incorporating the quality focus, and we created some specific initiatives aimed at the dissemination of the TQM agenda across the Health Centre. Meetings of key groups such as the Board, Management Committee, Medical Advisory Committee, and department managers' meetings are structured to allow a portion of time for reporting on the results of our quality efforts. New employee orientation now includes the introduction of total quality management; a new employee handbook emphasizes this focus. The underlying constancy of purpose, telling people we care and that what they do is important to our ability to serve the community, is a strong thread in our tapestry of success.

The Health Centre's publications — the weekly and monthly *Centre Report*, educational services' *Learning Matters,* and *Nursing Voice,* as well as the award-winning magazine NEXUS, and the Health Centre's annual report — regularly feature stories of successful projects, teamwork, and innovation. The communication in both picture and print of quality success stories was a priority right from the launch of St. Joseph's TQM initiative.

Other communications-oriented programs St. Joseph's created in the past few years are highly effective forums. Employee focus group lunches are held monthly and include open dialogue between frontline staff and me. The senior management and I also commit a portion of our time to attending regularly scheduled managers' breakfast meetings and to going on "rounds" with staff. My meetings with staff and managers on my walk-arounds or on more formal occasions focus on communicating the vision, the importance of staff, and the challenge of the changes we face.

We have also recently created a video library containing our vision video and other material relating to TQM, and there is a resource library that includes articles on TQM by St. Joseph's Health Centre staff and outside sources. TQM articles are regularly circulated to physicians and managers. It is important to provide them with articles that have insight into both the problem areas and success stories surrounding TQM.

Communications and staff training dynamically combine in the development across the Health Centre of a network of CQI training "graduates". Their meetings provide an effective forum for regular sharing of continuous quality improvement experiences, and also provide a natural setting for recognition. At each meeting, staff who have most recently completed CQI training receive graduation certificates, followed by the presentation of team results.

Creating lateral communications   There is one particularly crucial communications shift required by organizations intent on achieving total quality management. This is the need to develop strategies to accomplish *lateral communications*, which break down barriers between departments and areas. We are all familiar with top-down and bottom-up communications in the corporate world. Communicators have traditionally developed programs for making sure senior management stays in touch with the concerns and suggestions of grassroots staff. But with TQM comes a whole new dimension — communication across the various departments and functions of an organization.

Hospital staff are often not given information to understand the interdependence of the goals, responsibilities, and capabilities of other departments. To place this within the context of total quality management, the knowledge of other work groups becomes essential as we identify and improve cross-functional processes. If we are looking at patient flow, for example, how much easier it is to identify and find solutions to delays if each area already has a basic understanding of the other's role and function. It's a link from peer to peer, not the traditional employee-supervisor model.

The old employee-supervisor communications model was never a straight line. Communication usually went from employee through their supervisor to the manager, to the manager of a peer, and eventually down to another employee. Too often, the trail led to the vice-presidents and likely the CEO and then back down another trail. It is just this kind of hierarchy that impedes communication and decision-making. For hospital staff to be truly empowered, this process has to change.

In the Quality Climate Survey we asked staff about the reality of lateral communications on their jobs. Senior management then used this research data to help them understand how the lack of lateral communication affects quality. The Quality of Work Life Steering Committee and union presidents also became involved in setting up a new communications process for complex organizational change. Focus groups, management, and non-management provided input on obstacles and possible solutions. One idea being implemented across St. Joseph's is a series of interdepartmental visits in which one department invites their internal customers (another department) to its departmental meeting to talk about the services each provides the other and their mutual expectations.

Dealing with rumour and innuendo   A classic communications problem in most large organizations is the rumour mill. This means of communication typically creates misinformation or partial truths. At St. Joseph's we came to realize that, throughout all this change, people wanted more information and they wanted it more quickly than they were getting it.

Rumours were naturally part of the culture, yet they were causing some problems of accuracy and occasionally created unnecessary upset. As the organizational environment or external factors affected us, change was coming (and still is) rapidly. We decided to reverse the frustration traditionally expressed by management and chose to ask staff what they were hearing and to respond to these concerns. We now use daily (originally weekly) 30-60 second video messages called "Straight Talk" on well-placed monitors throughout the Health Centre. These messages simply confirm, deny, or clarify rumour which may be circulating among staff. The information is provided by the individual or department that is the "best source" for an accurate response to the issue.

I have taken the position, whether in these responses or at staff lunches or other encounters, that there are no secrets. Since coming to St. Joseph's, I can only think of two matters that required a high level of confidentiality — one was a major land acquisition and the other continues to be around private individual issues (for example, physician or other staff discipline, compensation, and so forth).

Nothing — including our budget or capital reserves, or information on how we spend our funds — is kept a secret. We have recently opened our Board meetings fully and will have *in camera* sessions only on a very exceptional basis. And to demystify the Board meetings and their processes, we have invited staff members to attend, especially union leaders.

Talking to the public   The free flow of information and effective communications processes within the Health Centre are important priorities at St. Joseph's. But no less crucial is the growing need for hospitals to improve the ways they communicate with the public. Patients and their families, as well as the community in general, want clear information about the many changes happening in the health care system, changes that affect their hospitals and the way they receive care. It is becoming more apparent through our patient surveys that people need to have the right to ask questions and to have them legitimized.

If, as I said in Chapter Two, we are indeed at the end of the era of hospitalization and making the transition to a system that will emphasize outpatient care, preventive health strategies, and more joint hospital-community initiatives, the public will increasingly demand to know what this system will look like and how it will care for the sick and injured.

Health care today is at the brink of a revolution. Communities across the nation are having to deal with new health care agendas of cost restraints coupled with the need to provide high quality services at reasonable cost. Hospitals can do a far better job of interpreting to the public what these changes mean to them, and how the hospitals and medical professionals themselves are adapting to difficult new realities. Through openness and integrity in their communications, hospitals must play a role in maintaining public confidence in health institutions and the health care system, despite the unsettledness of the times. The communication of health care issues to the public will have to go beyond just reporting news of medical breakthroughs or human interest stories of patients' experiences in hospitals. Instead, we must play a strong teaching role with communities on important issues such as health promotion, disease prevention, treatment outcomes, and the appropriate use of the health care system.

The hospital that believes TQM can recapture the current wasted resources — and I mean *wasted* — uses those gains to fashion a system that is more responsive to patients, offers a better working environment for staff, and delivers high quality care, must make its case in the public arena. Communications means more openness than thought possible. I believe that if you can't trust your staff, and if you cannot communicate well with them and the public you are serving, they cannot be expected to trust you or your organization — you haven't earned it.

Long-Term Evaluation The newness of total quality management to health care, and even to business and industry, makes it impossible at this point in time for anyone to say definitively that total quality management works in the long-term. Total quality management really only started to make inroads in certain U.S. hospitals in the mid-1980s, and in Canada, in the late 1980s. Yet some of the results thus far reported by the U.S.-based National Demonstration Project and a number of other American hospitals are impressive.

At a presentation on evaluation strategies for total quality management, Ross Baker, a professor in the department of health administration at the

University of Toronto, pointed to some of the outcomes achieved by quality improvement teams at the University of Michigan Medical Center as indicative of the direction of TQM. Improvements in operating-room efficiencies and volume saved $500,000 by eliminating unnecessary hospital stays. The achievement of decreased waiting times for admitted patients saved $200,000 in admitting costs, and reduction in the gap in time between a patient being judged ready for discharge and actually discharged saved $250,000.

The initial successes of total quality management at St. Joseph's Health Centre as well as similar outcomes at several other Canadian quality management pioneers, such as the University of Alberta Hospitals, Princess Margaret Hospital and Women's College Hospital in Toronto, the Freeport Hospital in Kitchener, Ontario, and the Victoria General in Halifax, Nova Scotia, offer early evidence of TQM's promise.

KEY COMPONENTS
HIGH LEVEL FLOW CHART
TQM Implementation Process

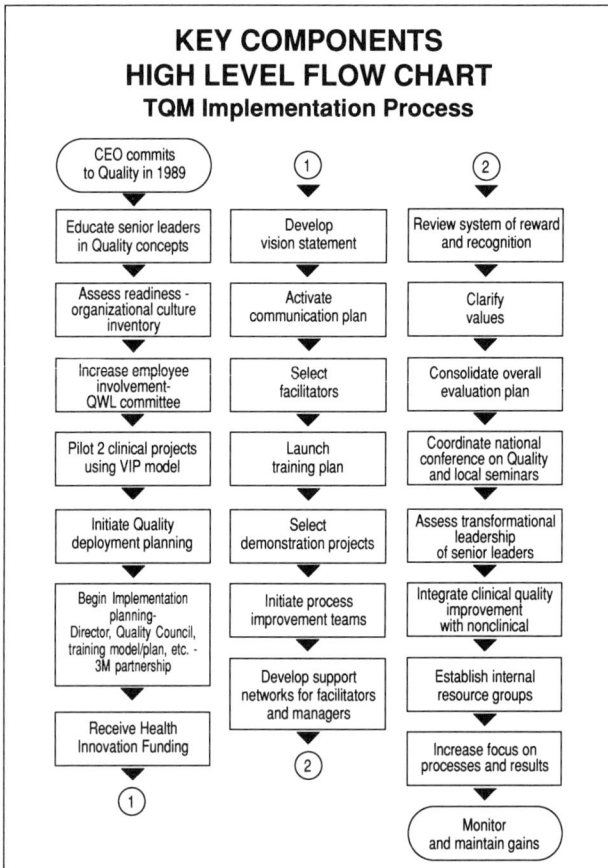

A vital strength of TQM is that it contains within itself the tools and methods to measure continually its own successes and shortcomings. It relies on the gathering of accurate and reliable data, as well as the stringent analysis of the results of the data and its impact on effecting change. While, at present, many of the successes of total quality management are often reported anecdotally, there is now a continual flow of evidence gradually building up through the work of continuous quality improvement teams, research projects, and senior management evaluations of organizational direction.

The data that has been collected, analysed, and used to create improvements in the system must also be used to help paint "the big picture." There must be a wide-ranging evaluation plan that addresses the need for more systematic research evidence on the effect of total quality management on health care organizations.

Included in the mandate of the Health Innovation fund awarded to St. Joseph's Health Centre by the Ministry of Health was that a portion of the money be used to develop an evaluation plan for total quality management in hospitals. In 1991, our hospital began a collaboration with the hospital-management research unit and others in the department of health administration at the University of Toronto. The evaluation plan was to look at changes at both the macro levels of the organization and the micro levels of CQI teams, and to include both quantitative and qualitative assessments.

The TQM evaluation plan developed at St. Joseph's in collaboration with the University of Toronto is organized to evaluate the key elements and issues associated with continuous improvement. In order to assess the long-term or lasting impact of continuous quality improvement teams, a major area of evaluation is team functioning, team effectiveness, team project outcomes, and the relationships between team activities and the continuous quality improvement pathway.

The tool St. Joseph's chose for the evaluation of teams is the extensive Team Meeting package developed by the University of Toronto's hospital-management research group. It includes ongoing records of team meetings during the life of specific improvement projects. There is a project worksheet to track activities, for example, from the teaching of CQI techniques to the implementation and evaluation of process improvements. The summary of the Team Meeting documents each meeting's specific agendas and the team's perceptions of the meeting's strengths and weaknesses. As well, each team member anonymously does an assessment of his or her impressions of the meeting and of the team's overall progress.

We also plan to do a post-project completion survey of the experience of CQI teams. However, in order to implement this evaluative tool, we must arrive at a consensus about what "completion" means. Is it when the team's implementation plan is complete? Or is it the time when the implementation plan has achieved the results the team planned for and can confidently demonstrate, thus sustaining the gains? The answer to these questions will influence the future development of CQI evaluative tools.

A second area of research is the ongoing evaluation of the organizational culture of St. Joseph's Health Centre — how far it has evolved into a culture of total quality management. With the assistance of the University of Toronto research team, St. Joseph's has developed a system of document review, including the mission statement, vision statement, and content of minutes of various key meetings. There is also a series of structured interviews with St. Joseph's senior management team to evaluate whether there is congruence between what they say and what they do. In addition, St. Joseph's is collaborating with the University of Western Ontario in the use of a tool, the Multifactor Leadership Questionnaire, to assess the development of Health Centre leaders toward transformational leadership.

The Transformational Leadership Development Program measures a broad variety of leadership styles ranging from passive leaders, to leaders who reward "followers," to those who are capable of transforming followers into leaders. Each senior leader indicates on the questionnaire how accurately he or she feels a series of adjectives describes his or her behaviour. A similar rating is performed by employees and colleagues who work with, or report to, the leader. The results of this tool will be used to help St. Joseph's senior team develop the motivational, inspirational, person-centred, and transformative qualities necessary to become astute and visionary leaders.

For St. Joseph's as a whole, the Organizational Culture Inventory of 1989-90 and the Quality Climate Survey of 1991 supplied base-line data. In the fall of 1992, we obtained some initial results of another survey tool, one developed by Development Dimensions International (DDI) and entitled "Barriers and Aids to Total Quality Management." The survey identifies some common themes supporting the success of total quality management at St. Joseph's. Among them are wide support and enthusiasm for CQI team efforts, awareness of senior management commitment, and an appreciation of the usefulness of continuous quality improvement techniques.

"I love the idea of CQI," wrote one staff member on the DDI survey. "It makes sense that the people who are most directly involved with the service would be the best people to pinpoint problem areas. Before, I would have an idea that made good sense to me but wouldn't voice it, because past experience showed that it might be well met, but nothing concrete would happen to implement it. Now if I have a suggestion, I run it by management and then try it out myself. Things are finally moving! Welcome to the 90s!"

"TQM means empowerment, open communication," wrote another. "The staff have taken the training and understand the concepts. They have a real desire to make it work. I feel best about the sharing of power."

Many staff mentioned the ability of the total quality management perspective to clarify customer satisfaction in terms of health care. "CQI is the first sensible system I have seen implemented in years," one person wrote, "We need to focus on our customers' needs. Their lives are in our hands."

But this survey's results do not allow us to rest on our laurels. Many persistent barriers to total quality continued to trouble staff. The pressure of funding restraints on the health care system, resulting in fewer staff and heavier workloads, was identified as a major concern. "There is never enough time to spend with each customer," wrote a staff member. "I like the statement 'walk the talk' but have not seen much as of yet."

Time commitment remains a formidable hurdle for many front-line staff and managers. "As the manager training the staff, it is very difficult to get employees away for sessions," a manager wrote. "There is no one to cover their area, and patient care must be the priority."

Other individuals identified time as a problem in the sense that they felt they had not had sufficient time to absorb the CQI training materials. Some mentioned that there were many in the Health Centre who were not yet convinced about CQI and some who were openly or covertly resistant.

Another aspect of St. Joseph's total quality management evaluation plan is the analysis of the costs of quality. This includes CQI implementation costs, prevention costs (costs incurred to prevent problems) such as training and development, patient education, and resource planning; appraisal costs (the costs of auditing and managing risk) such as quality assurance activities, utilization review, and charge auditing; and failure costs (costs of correcting failures and managing crisis), complications of medical procedures, multiple trips to hospital for repeat testing, potential loss of patient confidence in the hospital, and so forth.

The projects in clinical continuous quality improvement (CCQI) at St. Joseph's and at several other hospitals are useful in establishing a growing data base and an external benchmarking of case costs. As mentioned in Chapter Three, it is imperative that the health care system of the future be driven by successful treatment outcomes. We need to know what works and what doesn't.

And finally, the evaluation plan must have a major focus on customer satisfaction. This is a particularly important area for the evaluation of TQM in hospitals because it reveals the levels of patient satisfaction with the health care delivered to them and also addresses public perceptions of hospitals and health care.

A crucial factor to take into account in any evaluation process is that consideration of the prevention costs of quality must include attention to the development of realistic customer (patient) expectations. Total quality management data is used for more than gathering information on customer expectations. It must also be directed toward action plans that educate the public on which expectations of the system are realistic and which are not.

For example, it may be good service to succeed in reducing a physician's hospital clinic waiting time, say, by half an hour, but it would be unrealistic if patients identified good service as never having to wait more than five minutes. It will not be enough simply to exhort communities toward more understanding of the issues having significant impact on the health care system. The data provided by strategies of total quality management can be used to show the public what health care processes involve and how continuous improvements are being made.

The Angus Reid community survey provided us with enlightening information on how St. Joseph's is perceived by the community and on strongly held community values concerning health care. We have also developed several types of patient-satisfaction survey methods, including telephone surveys and written questionnaires. The total quality management approach aims for a health care system where the voice of the customer is as important as concerns about the economics and politics of health care.

The evaluation of the impact of total quality management must not simply remain in the realm of specific hospitals and individual communities, however. As more health institutions gain experience with continuous quality improvement techniques, there is a great need to share key learnings on a wider scale among hospitals, with governing bodies and with the general public as well.

When I review St. Joseph's efforts in total quality management with some organizations a few of the responses I get worry me. Some say, "We have been doing this for years." And I ask, "What have you really been doing?" The answer is usually something along the lines of, "Improving what we do." And of course, I get examples.

What may be lacking is the commitment to the systemic transformation of the organization. Or perhaps the identified changes are totally driven from above with little input from staff. In spite of the importance of organizational integrity and occasional CEO ego, there is little evidence I can find that they are creating the breadth of structures, processes, and results necessary for dynamic viability in the next decade and beyond.

At the October 1992 "Owning the Future" conference, Ross Baker identified several key questions that need organizational researchers' and health care analysts' attention in order to obtain answers that move, as Baker puts it, "out of the realm of opinion" toward accurate measurement of principles and strategies. He summarized these key research questions as: Are particular types of organizational culture more receptive to CQI? How does CQI affect organizational culture? Are there patterns in the ways an organization implementing CQI changes its culture? Is cultural change a prerequisite for successful CQI teamwork in an organization? And finally: Is cultural change a requirement for making CQI part of the fabric of the organization?

These are important questions and will no doubt keep organizational researchers busy for some years to come. But such is the urgency of the need for change in the health care system, and particularly in hospitals, that we cannot afford to wait until all the answers are in.

7

The New Health Care Leader

The wicked leader is he who the people despise.
The good leader is he who the people revere.
The great leader is he who the people say
"We did it ourselves."

— LAO TSU

Never has the issue of leadership in health care been more critical than it is today. Many hospital administrators feel they are increasingly in a no-win situation, desperately caught up in trying to cut costs and keep their hospitals within their allotted budgets while continuing to manage using established models and methods. It is time for health care administrators to stop thinking of themselves only in terms of their administrative functions and instead make the decision to become leaders.

The problems and challenges of our health care systems need more than analysis and impassioned calls for change. They need action. Leadership will either move health care into the future or will be the bane of the system's, and its hospitals', existence. Health care management generally, across much of North America, is at a stalemate. Yesterday's management styles and strategies are not working. Hospital staff — both medical and nonmedical — have turned to senior management for leadership and have been disappointed. Content to try to keep abreast of government policy directions and funding admonitions, or to navigate with difficulty the stormy waters of agendas and power struggles among medical professionals, other hospitals, government, unions, and communities, leaders in our hospitals have failed to lead.

THE NEW DEFINITION OF LEADERSHIP

Now, on the threshold of the twenty-first century, leadership must be defined as something substantially different from what it was in previous decades. It can no longer be framed in terms of unquestioned authority and power. Dramatic events worldwide paint another picture. The spirit of democracy and self-determination has swept with cataclysmic energy throughout countries of the former eastern bloc. Angry crowds, demoralized by poverty and enraged by systemic racism, rioted and looted Los Angeles streets in the spring of 1992. And the normally even-tempered Canadian public has on an increasing number of occasions taken to firing off bitter invective at their elected politicians, federal and provincial.

Leaders of the future in health care and virtually every other industry, business, social service, and government ministry will be required to understand customer needs, gauge the effect of what they do to meet these needs, improve processes, develop and invest in people, and lead with vision. Leadership by fiat will not work, nor will an administrative approach that takes the form of avoidance, hiding behind policies, or ignoring pressing or controversial issues in the hope that problems will just go away.

Without a new type of leadership, hospitals will be unable to meet the demands of tomorrow — both from a medical and management perspective. Poorly led hospitals will not attract the finest medical talent, nor will they be readily able to move in new program direction. The consumers of health care — patients — increasingly are demanding accountability from hospitals, that the medical services offered be the best available, and that health care institutions use tight tax dollars wisely.

Hospital administrators trapped in the traditional mode of managers devising management policies and guidelines, supervisors enforcing the policies and guidelines, and front-line workers carrying them out, will not be able to transform their hospitals to meet the needs of consumers and health care service providers. Much of the difficulty involved in transforming our current management inadequacies into leadership strengths lies in the nature of widely held perceptions of health care itself.

Organizational consultant Ian Percy, who has worked with over 100 hospitals on creating management strategies and a vision for the future, talks about what he calls the "pathology of the business of medicine." Health care administrators are drawn to lead our institutions the same way we do medicine in our society. Every issue is a problem to be "diagnosed." Relationships externally with patients, governments, and communities are problem-based; so are relationships internally among hospital staff.

The effect of much medical care in the late twentieth century, observes Percy, has been the creation of powerful dependencies. "Just think of what happens when you enter hospital as a patient. Your belongings are taken from you, you are assigned a room, and you put on a nondescript hospital gown. The treatment you are going to receive is explained to you and you are prepped for the procedure, but something in you is also aware that your well-being, your very survival, is in the hands of medical professionals. *They* know how to handle the problem; *you* do not." The system must become patient-centred, refocused to providing more control by the patient — far greater than we have yet to see.

It is difficult to think of the future in terms of preventive health strategies or proactive health care management initiatives when you are caught up in a problem-based diagnostic model. People in the business of health promotion, who are involved in trying to develop community health strategies, often express the view that the greatest obstacle to preventive, community-based health care is the dominance of the medical model itself — the organization of the health care system primarily around illness and crisis.

Percy believes many of the calls for change, new strategies, and more effective direction in health care arise not from any real vision of what the future could be, but from the "pain" in today's health care system. The situation is clearly getting uncomfortable, as funding resources dwindle and waiting lists get longer. Pressures are mounting, and so we search frantically for avenues of constructive change. Pain and discomfort may well push us in the direction of seeing the need for change, but without a dream of the future — a picture of where we want to go — we will not be able, in meeting the health care needs of the next century, to accomplish the transformation our hospitals require to maintain the intent of the Canada Hospital Act, which ensures the system remains universally accessible, comprehensive, and publicly administered.

When Percy first began consulting with St. Joseph's Health Centre, he did so recognizing the opportunity to work with an organization determined to be focused on creating a better vision for the future rather than remaining in a "problem" orientation. "We need to understand what we are really dealing with," he says. "It's not just a matter of trying to 'walk the talk,' as the buzzword phrase goes these days. Something has to happen inside. Ten years ago, it was not acceptable in organizational circles to talk about the concept of 'spiritual leadership,' but that is exactly what many people today in positions of authority are struggling with and trying to articulate. They want a way of leadership that comes out of an inner conviction that what they are doing is worthwhile and that it will accomplish some good."

This type of leadership is not one of aggression, nor of the best-articulated policy position, nor of the most technical, scientific knowledge, but one of moral integrity rooted in deeply held human values. If the vision for our hospitals is that they be organizations practising total quality in everything they do, then our leaders must awaken in others the thirst for doing the same thing with their lives.

Warren Bennis, in his book *On Becoming A Leader*, has observed that "the ingredients of leadership cannot be taught . . . they must be learned." Leadership and the quest for quality are not something "taught" by management agendas and the content of seminars. They are learned by people who begin to engage not only their head but also their heart in the smallest task to the most complex.

The health care leader of the future will not rule but serve. People are tired of self-serving managers, CEOs, and politicians. In fact, the idea of service, whether framed in the concept of serving customers well in the marketplace or in the larger context of benefiting society, is central to economic, political, and social realities as they are unfolding today. In North America, over a very short period of time, we have seen our economy move from an industrial base to a service base. The thousands of jobs lost in the manufacturing sector and among the semiskilled labour force will not likely be gained back. Economists now estimate that two-thirds of our economy will be service-based. If this is true, we will need to manage with vastly different skills than we had in the past.

Bennis provides good insight into the characteristics of true leaders. Included are guiding vision, passion, integrity, and curiosity. The days of the charismatic personality, the hero in times of crisis, are over. That kind of leader may have created a powerful image of self, or even a powerful image of power, but often did not create an atmosphere or culture that motivated others toward positive long-term change; the management atmosphere often reflected needs for immediate results, a state of affairs symbolic of the illnesses in many organizations today.

Today's health care leaders must profoundly reconsider the way they function, their role, and the value they add to hospitals. Some of the knowledge gained in the past, along with certain skills and abilities, have led to management behaviours that are clearly no longer equal to the demands today's hospitals are placing upon those who must lead them. What we know about how to run organizations today will not help us tomorrow.

A first and crucial step for health care leaders in seeing themselves as there to serve rather than as high-powered administrators dominating a complex bureaucracy is to rethink the power trip some perpetuate both within and outside the hospital environment. They must admit to themselves and to their institutions that they have become part of the problem in fostering the organizational dependencies and barriers that impede both true leadership and functional quality. "If the organization is not growing, the leader is in the way," Percy says bluntly. Growing is no longer quantitative. The organization asserts the need for qualitative growth, and thus, the total quality movement.

Hospital administrators and medical professionals easily fall prey to the enormous busyness of the medical environment. Day-to-day events are so demanding, complex, and time-consuming that these individuals soon readily believe that things cannot happen without them. But how much of this truly serves the customers — patients and internal hospital staff — and how much of it is there to justify the existence of the administrator and the administrative structures?

The folly of this sort of leadership became so evident to me on a visit to Argentina. The deputy minister of the province of Buenos Aires believed the system of hospitals could not run without his direct involvement. The province encompasses many millions of people. At one point, all cases of measles were being reported to him so that he could "manage" the effect such an outbreak would have on hospitals. For what purpose, I could never determine.

We in administration create similar problems by thinking that if we have information about every issue, we can control the system we think we own. And hospital boards have been complicit in expecting CEOs to know everything about what is going on in the organization. We fall victim to every question and potential problem, and so provide answers to often minor problems that are better handled at other levels, particularly if the staff is clear on the vision, values, and goals of the institution, and functions within that framework.

A similar challenge confronts the practice of medicine itself. More knowledgeable and informed patients, stronger demands for medical accountability, and less respect for authority in general, are assailing the old authoritarian, paternalistic model of medicine based on "doctor knows best." Slowly we have been seeing medicine move toward the concept of shared care, and the articulation of ethical standards surrounding such issues as informed consent and quality of life has become a key consideration in treatment decisions.

The organizational tools of the past, based on the assumption of the "normalcy" of hierarchical structure, which for western civilization had its roots in Greco-Roman, Egyptian, and Judaeo-Christian antiquity, are not capable of responding adequately to today's economic, political, social, and health care complexities. Organizational visionaries looking for the seeds of a new leadership model find a more fitting metaphor in the realm of quantum science, with its premise that everything that happens influences and alters everything else in the field, and that energy is never destroyed, only redirected or transformed. Hospital systems need to evolve away from hierarchy toward a multi-dimensional, fluid, and seamless pattern of delivering health care responsive to individual needs.

LEADERS AND VISION

In his book Bennis presents several key themes, but most compelling is his discussion on being visionary in a way that "lifts people out of their petty preoccupations." It is the ability to see beyond the immediate term and to articulate the future or "manage the dream." Is not the hallmark of a great leader the ability to provide people with the sense of a dream that is not only achievable, but which also stretches people beyond their present capacities?

As a leader, you cannot take people farther than where you are yourself. And so the challenge for the leader is threefold — to create a vision so worthy you simply have to go there, to foster an environment where "visioning" is encouraged, and finally to translate vision to action. Futurist Joel Barker poetically expresses the vision/action dynamic as:

Vision without action is merely a dream.
Action without vision just passes the time.
Vision with action can change the world.[1]

Vision means precisely what the word implies — seeing. So many corporate executives, hospital CEOs among them, are very adept at analysis and at developing policies, guidelines, and strategies. But the skill needed for vision is one hardly ever taught in business administration programs: the development of the human imagination, the capacity to use imagery to create dramatic and vivid pictures of the organizations and workplaces we want for our society now and in the future. Many athletes, artists, and performers use mental imagery and mental rehearsal to help hone their skills and achieve their goals. Imaging and visioning are not esoteric New Age practices, but powerful creative tools.

Gareth Morgan, the author of *Images of Organization,* recently spoke to a group of us about some of his ideas and concepts of using imagery to create new solutions from inside ourselves, as opposed to externally, or borrowing from other organizations. He used the image of how a spider plant shoots off new spider plants to illustrate how we can begin looking at ways in which the organization may need to be shaped for the future. Each one of those plants are tied by a plenum, or umbilical cord, to the main plant. Morgan spoke of why spider plants shoot these off. Often it is when they are root bound — which gives us maybe another clue as to what the problem is with large, complex organizations, and how we must look at them as sprouting off and developing the small individual work units that are part of the whole and connected to it. The question is: What is that connection? What should it constitute? In the case of spider plant, it initially provides nourishment to the smaller plants, it has created. And if the shoots land on soil, they become self-sustaining and the plenum dies. The question really is: Does this give us some vital new ideas on how organizations might look in the future? This is but one example of the kind of work Morgan is doing and perhaps is the kind of creativity through images that we need to appreciate, understand, and look beyond the traditional viewpoint of organizations.

Today's leaders need to allow themselves to dream, to be able to imagine the new, unconcerned with whether it is possible under current policies or in the face of certain problems. Nothing kills a dream faster than questions such as: "Where will we find the room for this new program?";

"How much will it cost?"; "What if we try it and it doesn't work?"; or, "I talked with John Smith over at hospital X and he says they tried something like that last year but it didn't have the results they'd hoped for."

The time to consider practicalities or to seek advice is after you have done your visioning. If you cannot first see in your imagination what it is you want to create, you will lose your way once you encounter all the complexities, obstacles, and challenges on the road to making the vision become reality.

Visioning takes the leader from the realm of daily "rational" organizational tasks into the play of creativity. When you paint the picture of the ideal hospital, or most importantly, the ideal health care system, you can invoke the creative play of imagination by assuming that the reality you currently see is neither true nor false. Assume that every "high pain" hassle is reversible — that patients will not be kept waiting for long periods of time, that X-rays will never be misplaced, that only those medical tests absolutely necessary for the patient will be done, that hospital food will always be delicious, and so forth.

For health care organizations, the achievement of total quality management means creating a vision that breaks out of the old paradigm. Total quality management in health care means not only streamlining processes, but expanding the minds of care providers, management, and support staff to alter the way they do their work, expressing a vision within the context of a hospital's fundamental values to enable them to change their way of thinking or to look at what they do in relation to the larger community served. To be visionaries, leaders must be passionate about creating the culture of quality throughout the organization. A vision for the future of our hospitals must be more than a model that solves problems; it must also excite people. If staff, patients, and communities cannot believe in the future depicted for the hospital, it will be impossible to focus energy to achieve that vision.

This is hard work. We hear people talk about "working smarter, not harder." But the fact remains: this is not about physical work but about mental effort; it is a muscle that needs to be exercised in the workplace. It is extremely difficult for those who have not used the creative part of their mind to begin to do so in the midst of so much pressure and change. It is essential to consider ways to stimulate the creation of imagery that can extend into a vision, and then to make it a vision shared by others. Work by Edward De Bono and others in the area of human creativity, thinking, and imagination, has shown us that it is possible to learn new ways of thinking, ways that are very creative in nature.

Many times we, as CEOs, have not only repressed our own creative spirit, but have overtly stymied the creative thinking of those around us, colleagues and co-workers who have relied on us for organizational direction. We have not been comfortable outside the technical, scientific, logical arena. What we must do is become capable of generating imaginative new ideas and give others the time and inclination to do the same.

Forms of Total Quality Management in the Marketplace Today The move toward total quality management in business and industry, and increasingly in health care, has tended to be described in the marketplace in three forms. The first is the growing recognition, due to the profusion of magazine articles and numerous conferences, of such phrases as "continuous quality improvement" and "total quality management"; they have become hot. Some organizations have decided to "adopt CQI" because the business press has made it trendy. Or they have seen others succeeding at it, but themselves do not have leaders in the organization with a fundamental passionate commitment. This approach is almost certainly destined to fail.

The second form quality initiatives take in organizations is a programmatic one. It works this way: there is some understanding in the organization of the principles of quality and of the need for learning new ways of managing and leading to achieve quality, and so the organization starts training programs and sets up quality projects involving "work teams" to analyse work processes and come up with suggestions for improvement. While better than the trend-driven, lip-service approach, this path is also likely doomed to failure because total quality management cannot happen only as a result of courses followed by a series of activities.

While looking closely at work processes is a key tool of continuous quality improvement, the focus of such activities should always be on concrete outcomes. People working on quality projects must have a specific goal in mind, as well as the tools to measure whether the outcome is being accomplished. For example, if a hospital project team in the emergency department at St. Joseph's Health Centre decides to analyse the reasons patients are kept waiting for hours before receiving medical attention, it then must come up with a specific goal, such as "reduce the average three-hour waiting time to forty minutes," create strategies to accomplish the goal, and use solid data to measure both success and reasons for failure.

This represents a type of breakthrough thinking in health care. Breakthrough thinking is to *create* the vision of what customers think are the most important processes and outcomes for their care and then to strive for it. This requires thinking that stretches our present-day reality and very likely will disintegrate the very assumptions that encumber us and form barriers to potentially major changes of the sort that can significantly improve our services to patients and staff alike.

At St. Joseph's, for instance, the hematology and kidney (renal dialysis) unit realized that it took more than one and a half hours from the decision to obtain a blood sample to the time when its results were available on the unit for the physician to determine a clinical action. Now, it is in the order of one and a half *minutes* to obtain these results. For this group, this is breakthrough thinking in action. For the hospital as a whole, our 1993 strategic quality plan will be our first attempt to achieve breakthrough thinking — and thus results — in a few major processes, such as the complete admitting-discharge process.

Indeed, the third way is the only successful pathway for total quality management to sustain itself in the organization, one that settles for nothing less than the substantial transformation of the organizational culture from the CEO through to all staff. It links quality to the organizational values and helps the organization further refine these values toward a service, rather than institutional focus. It also definitively links process analysis and values with concrete results. In other words, it is a vision with the ability to achieve itself.

The organization must become a culture of change, and of learning to manage change, in the direction of better and better service through projects and activities that achieve measurable outcomes. It has one constancy of purpose, and that is the inalienable needs of the patients.

Implicit in leadership is risk. Change creates a sense of uncertainty. As Deming says, the leader must sustain the constancy of purpose while the organization realigns itself through a TQM strategy. Uncertainty, confusion, and anxiety will inevitably accompany any significant change, and the short-term reaction of administrators may be to attempt to provide a heroic quick fix to any stress or chaos, or alternatively, to give up.

In the past year, several articles in popular publications, including the *Harvard Business Review* and *Newsweek*, have indicated disenchantment

with the results of total quality management in some American corporations. Where total quality initiatives have failed, or delivered less than
successful results, these articles cite getting wrapped up in "activities" and
processes without regard for outcome, and expecting "instant gratifica-
tion" from TQM, as major factors in the failure of total quality management to take hold in an organization. "Of course," comment *Newsweek*
writers Jay Mathews and Peter Katel, "a handful of companies, like Xerox,
Motorola, Federal Express, and Harley-Davidson, have made TQM work,
partly because such firms have the patience advocates say is essential. But
such companies are exceptions in an American climate where management plans often have the shelf life of cottage cheese."[2]

Within hospitals there are similar dangers, in fact more likely so.
Dramatic new developments in medicine and science, the rapidity of
change in health care environments, and the presence of powerful high
technology in hospitals have led to a perception in the minds of many that
the very nature of medicine calls for it to deliver a quick fix for what ails
us. When we are ill and in need of treatment, we want answers immediately. The relentlessly fast pace of modern hospitals makes the
patience, determination, and vision to achieve organizational transformation difficult to sustain.

In an interview for the magazine *Hospitals* in June 1992, Donald
Berwick observed that skeptics' questions must be taken seriously and
that hospitals intent on achieving total quality must not lose their quality-
oriented vision.

> In some ways, the questions are on target; the reason to do this is to
> achieve unprecedented levels of care and outcome and cost results.
> Until that's happened, there will be skeptics. . . . We really need to
> do something that's better and different for our patients. You don't
> get there by moving water coolers. You have to have a vision, an
> overarching systemic view . . . So quality management's a method,
> but it doesn't tell you what to do with the method. What we've got to
> do is use the method to make a much better system. We've still got
> to reach for that level of vision.[3]

LEADERS AND INTEGRITY

As Bennis so aptly observes in *On Becoming A Leader*, the leader with
integrity possesses self-knowledge, candour, and maturity. Trust is central

to integrity. Promises and commitments must be kept, and among people who work in the organization there is a sense of honour. Reliability and consistency are key characteristics of a leader who is trying to implement total quality management. The reliability and consistency of the core values articulated by the leader provide stability during the extended period of change needed to transform the organization to a culture of total quality management.

One major element leading to the failure of TQM strategies in the industrial sector is the inability of many workplaces to get beyond the us versus them barrier typical not only of union-management relations, but also of the relationship between senior management and middle management, and middle management and front-line staff. Good intentions and high-sounding phrases are not enough; many workers, in hospitals as much as anywhere else, are cynical of management platitudes about teamwork and employee participation. Well, it is imperative we go far beyond even these notions.

Just as the visionary function of leadership must be tied to concrete results, so too must the integrity of "walking the talk" of quality be linked to desired outcomes. There must be a sense in the organization that those in positions of leadership, who have the responsibility for setting the direction of the future, *mean* what they say and are committed to the values inherent in the vision they are espousing.

Health care is particularly vulnerable to the us versus them mentality because many hospitals, in addition to having employees who are unionized and with whom hospital management must negotiate collective agreements, also have within their walls numerous individuals and departments with high levels of education and highly specialized skills. Every hospital, large or small, contends daily not only with the demands of patient care, but with a large number of professional agendas among its staff.

The relationship of physicians with hospital management also adds a complex dimension. Hospital administrators can be at odds with physicians, and vice versa, over management issues and decisions concerning the policies and direction of the hospital's many care programs. The inclusion of physicians as key health care system stakeholders in total quality management must go beyond platitudes to workable partnerships that support the values and practices of total quality. More time and effort must be made with physicians, as discussed in Chapter Three, so that they understand the organization's vision and the part they play.

A hospital CEO, medical chief of staff, or other senior management personnel, cannot be all things to all people in an environment as diverse as a hospital. But the one thing they *can* communicate consistently is their integrity, that they do have a strong commitment to quality, and that they value the contribution of people and their skills to the organization.

LEADERS AND LEARNING

Peter Senge characterizes future-oriented leaders as those who have a relentless commitment to learning along with the strength to resolve past issues and develop confidence in themselves and in others. In order to become better at what they do, leaders must unlearn some of their most basic management attitudes. Whether the orientation of how to deal with current reality and of how to make our environment predictable and relatively secure was learned early from parents or later from traditional management education in universities, we need now to cast it aside. The old way of managing through controlling, planning, and organizing simply continues to reinforce within the organization the classic parent-child relationship.

Today's leaders must, in a management sense, be prepared to give up their parental role, which generates below-the-surface dependencies. In the same way, physicians are moving away from the paternalistic practice patterns of the past toward models of care that include patients in treatment decision-making. Relinquishing the parental role means that leaders in organizations have to be willing to allow their workforce to function as responsible adults. They have to trust people to do their jobs.

But even more importantly, leaders must reawaken in people a desire for continuous learning. Implementing TQM requires establishing, or re-establishing, an unquenchable thirst for learning throughout the organization. This is no small task, because most adults today, including corporate and institutional CEOs, are the products of an educational system that emphasized content, competition, the regurgitation of fact-based material, and a teacher-driven learning agenda. One of the most important challenges facing North American school boards, colleges, and universities is the reframing of educational systems to better prepare individuals to function successfully in today's global marketplace.

Because of the proliferation of knowledge in this latter half of the twentieth century, no longer is it possible to *know* everything about a subject. The amount of available medical knowledge is ever increasing, and many other professions and skill-based occupations face similar knowledge acceleration. What we now need are not individuals who are adept at memorizing content, but individuals who know how to learn. Much of the future focus of educational programs will be not in providing definitive answers, but in teaching people how to go about discovering what it is they need to know. Every faculty of medicine in Canada now has adopted, or shortly will have, the learner-centred model of education in place of the old traditional approach.

Leaders must remove the albatrosses around their necks and address their need to "know it all," so that they become more the servant of their organizations and less self-serving. Many procedures, policy guidelines, and strategy plans exist as much for management control and reasons of power and status as they do for furthering the work of the organization (and as anyone who has ever worked in health care can attest, such paper-driven activities are rampant). While policies and guidelines provide parameters for making choices, certainly in health care, from a total quality management perspective they, too, must be tied to outcomes. Do their outcomes serve and empower the customer and the worker, or merely stroke the self-importance of the executive officer or manager and get in the way of constructive results?

We cannot continue to be trapped by our past. Warren Bennis observes, "All the leaders I talked with agreed that no one can teach you how to become yourself, to take charge, to express yourself, except you."4 By the time we reach puberty, Bennis says, we have been shaped by family, friends, school, and society to a far greater extent than we realize. We have been told how to be. "But people begin to become leaders at the moment when they decide for themselves how to be . . . rather than being designed by your experience, you become your own designer. You become cause *and* effect rather than mere effect, . . . You make your life your own by understanding it."5

The "leader as servant" models the customer-centred imperative. This form of leadership helps the organization achieve the systemic changes required to implement total quality management. We leaders of hospitals must understand the basic changes in behaviour necessary for us to be seen as part of the solution. We must accept and come to terms with our vulnerability and expose it as part of the change necessary for our transformation.

A large part of leadership, in encouraging what Senge calls "generative learning," is striving to enlarge the learning circle throughout the entire organization. Such concepts as mentoring, cross-functional teams, and collaborative decision-making become second nature to a leader intent on expanding the circle of learning and generating the energy that a desire for continuous learning engenders in such an environment.

Our hospitals contain the potential for sharing a lot of learning among staff, and for broadening learning circles that ultimately will better serve patients. Unfortunately, the fact that most hospitals have been designed along departmental lines works against this. It is one of the great strengths of total quality management and strategies of continuous quality improvement that departmental boundaries can become more fluid as quality solutions are sought across departments, not simply within them.

The expansion of learning circles should go beyond the individual hospital, too. The potential for sharing key learnings and quality strategies with other health institutions and with other types of care givers, both nationally and internationally, has not really been explored, much less attempted (except in medical research). It is time for hospitals to end their competitiveness and territoriality. Instead, they should regard one another as collaborators in acquiring health care knowledge and skills, and delivering service to communities. Community agencies involved in health must be part of the bigger, more relevant learning circles.

LEADERS AND CHANGE

Mastering change to transform an organization begins with a reassessment of self and a deepening understanding of the changing demands of customers, both internal and external. In order for change not to descend into chaos or simply become a program of change for change's sake, it must be grounded in the intrinsic value of persons and their right to compassionate and competent medical care when they are ill.

An understanding of why change is imperative is vital. What is different about today and tomorrow? Why will today's practices — in our hospitals and in business and industry — not work tomorrow? If the reality of change and the reasons change is happening are not clearly expressed, both within the organization and to the public in general, staff become cynical and unable to focus on the future, and the public becomes cynical about the ability of the organization to serve them. At each level of the organization, people must be given more opportunity to use their skills;

this enables organizations to become more powerful in solving problems and achieving their visions.

Since about the mid-1980s, the word "empowerment" has been thrown around business circles ad nauseam. Many in the workforce, including hospital staff, have become understandably distrustful and skeptical of the term, often seeing it as a management ploy to manipulate them into taking on increasing responsibilities without increasing salaries or giving adequate recognition. Others see "empowerment" as abdicating responsibility entirely to others, letting others do it, and not having to be accountable for the results. During the strike by Cami Automotive workers in fall 1992, the workers claimed that "participative management" and "empowerment" meant that they had to take on management's responsibilities.[6]

The misunderstandings and widespread confusion over what the concept means are no doubt major factors in why empowerment in the workplace often fails and why people get discouraged. Empowerment is not something one person gives another. Seeing it in this perspective perpetuates the us-versus-them dichotomy — empowerment as something senior management bestow upon each other and their staff. But real empowerment is the ability to identify and remove the barriers in the system that prevent the expression of personal excellence or the development of improvement and innovation in both individuals and the organization.

Empowerment in this sense requires a fundamental reorientation of those who lead, and it is at the heart and soul of total quality management. Not only at the senior level must leadership be operative, it must be apparent at *every* level; a major characteristic of empowerment is that it helps key individuals within the organization become leaders, simultaneously removing the barriers that keep them from exercising their leadership.

The notion that, in hospitals, senior administrators, physicians, or other powerful professional groupings control others must be shaken to its roots and replaced with an understanding that, given the right goals, the right information, the right skills, and working within agreed upon values, the organization will succeed because of the collective efforts of individuals. Even the word "management" may gradually fall out of use. At St. Joseph's, the managers have come to realize the inadequacy of their title. Their role is changing such that managing people is no longer the primary way we achieve our goals; rather, it is through empowering and coaching them.

A new way of leading and empowering others also implies a change in hiring practices within organizations. Leaders will seek to hire individuals who not only have the best skills for the job but whose minds and hearts are open to the vision and commitment demanded by a culture of total quality management.

In health care, the concepts of empowerment and embracing change apply not only to medical professionals, related medical disciplines, and health care service providers working within hospitals and community health agencies, but directly to communities. Such leadership will be in the form of well-developed patient education programs, public awareness of health care issues, and a clearer focus on the role of health promotion within the health care system.

More importantly, as we shift care to the community, hospitals must focus less inwardly and more outwardly, looking beyond their walls and seeing the potential advantages of health care delivery in ways that stretch our previous thinking. Further, the community must understand the issues and create its own priorities for health. No amount of specialty care for those close to death has significantly improved the health status of the *community*. Only surfactant, a substance that came into use in the 1980s to assist in the maturing of the lungs of premature infants, has appreciably added to the statistical lengthening of life for Canadians.

Another complex arena of change are hospital boards. There is an increasingly prevalent perception that leadership in hospitals must come, first and foremost, from the board. In Ontario, proposed changes to the Public Hospitals Act have focused on a rather heated debate on who should be on hospital boards. The feeling by some that board members should be elected or appointed rather than voluntary is likely based in the desire of communities to have their interests truly represented. But there is no evidence at this point that such newly constituted hospital boards will do a better job than the existing voluntary ones. Hospitals across Canada are dealing with similar thorny issues of governance, and provincial governments are increasingly looking at structural changes in the direction of regionalization of health care services. The governance issue in Canadian health care will be a major focus of health care policy direction for some time to come, and will require strong, articulate, visionary leadership to arrive at a solution that does not compromise quality.

Those who do make up the membership of hospital boards in the new health care and organizational climate will need to understand and promote the changing roles and evolving expectations of the CEO and staff. No longer can they expect the CEO to understand and offer solutions to problems occurring at every level of the hospital. Rather, the fundamental responsibility of the CEO is creating strategic direction, communicating the vision, maintaining the values, and implementing policy. It is the CEO who must create the passion and enthusiasm of the vision so that others will become committed.

Hospital boards and CEOs, as leaders in total quality management, will have to understand accountability as being achieved through demonstrated commitment to improving systems that serve customers — patients and hospital staff — and through reaching mutually agreed upon goals aligned with the values of the hospital and of health care in general. From the board room to senior management to medical staff to nonmedical staff, a hospital is created that is change-oriented, whose staff understands the reasons for change — thus substantially eliminating cynicism — and takes ownership to make the vision of the future a reality.

LEADERSHIP AND COMMUNICATION

Total quality management depends on a leader who enables others to understand the needs of external customers and who motivates the internal improvements necessary to meet or exceed their needs. The leader involved with change must be a supreme communicator. He or she must communicate with staff to ensure that together they understand both the process and the results of what they are aiming to accomplish. Open, receptive communication provides the stability and consistency they will need for what, in effect, is a journey of continuous change. Everyone within the organization is a partner in creating the communications network so that every area understands the other, and care and service to customers is improved. Effective communication is a clear indication of the degree of unity within the organization. There can be no secrets — even risking uncertainty may be the only way to have many within the organization own the agenda of needed changes.

Hospitals themselves are communities; indeed, in some of the larger health complexes the number of employees is as large as many North American small towns. They are communities of healing, without question, but they are also communities where people eat together, work, argue, collaborate, laugh, cry, grow tired, respond to crisis, and where staff often go the extra distance for their patients and each other. Burnout occurs especially when someone gives too much and gets back too little. This is why communication is so valuable, particularly the recognition of what people are doing and struggling with at every level of the organization.

The seamless health care system with no service or communication breakdowns among hospitals, community agencies, physicians, government, and patients may well evolve from the creation of quality health institutions that foster a sense of connectedness among their staff and a corresponding connectedness with patients. It has been said of total quality management that one of its greatest strengths is that it gives people the sense of being part of something, connected to each other and to the overarching vision of the organization.

"Bridging the Leadership Gap," a study conducted by Kodak and Healthcare Forum published in May 1992, notes that mastering change, continuous quality improvement, and systems thinking are major discrepancies between the current and future practices of health care leaders. In other words, we have hardly begun — and we had better get going.

Health care needs leaders who will inspire, liberate, and create an atmosphere that motivates health care teams toward new understanding. Health care leaders must stop using traditional paradigms and become willing to change their behaviour. There is no question that our health care system today calls out for leaders who are fit mentally, emotionally, spiritually, and physically. As Joel Barker says, leaders lead between paradigms; managers manage within them. The concepts of total quality management and their application to health care require much more than intellectual understanding and good intentions. They require the ability to live the vision, so that people see and feel the expression of these values in everything a leader says and does.

8

"The Road Less Travelled": Hospital CEOs in Roundtable Discussion

Two roads diverged in a wood, and I — I took the one less travelled by. And that has made all the difference.

— ROBERT FROST

A number of Canadian hospitals have begun the quality journey, propelled by the same urgency as St. Joseph's to address the health care crisis and the far-reaching changes necessary to assure our patients high-quality medical care now and in the future. Total quality in health care needs to move from individual, hospital-based initiatives to a national health care focus. At the October 1992 "Owning the Future" forum, I met some of my colleagues from other hospitals for lunch. I wanted to hear their views on the need for change in the Canadian health care system, their experience with total quality management thus far, and their perceptions about the ability of total quality management to guide those changes.

Joining me at the table were Donald Schurman, president of University of Alberta Hospitals in Edmonton, Alberta; Dr. Donald Carlow, president and CEO of the Ontario Cancer Institute/Princess Margaret Hospital in Toronto, Ontario; Dr. Bernard Badley, president and CEO of Victoria General Hospital in Halifax, Nova Scotia; and Patricia Henderson, executive director of the Freeport Hospital, a chronic/rehabilitation hospital in Kitchener-Waterloo, Ontario.

These individuals are among the as yet small group of total quality management pioneers in Canada. The health care institutions they serve are in various stages of implementing TQM. Organizational consultant Ian Percy kept the discussion moving with some leading questions. I deliberately played a low-key role so that this chapter would reflect the views of other health care leaders. We were also joined for part of the discussion by Sister Mary Jean Ryan, the president and CEO of the Sisters of St. Mary Health Care System. She was one of the forum's keynote speakers and reminded us that both sides of the border have much in common on the journey toward transforming health care.

In your opinion, what is "quality" in health care?

Donald Schurman: I think my definition of quality in health care would be provision of effective services on a timely basis in a fashion that's satisfying to the patients, at a cost that society can afford.

Isn't that what we've been saying in health care for a very long time?

Schurman: It isn't. It's very different. We've never talked about measurements of effectiveness. We haven't talked very much about costs. We haven't talked very much about satisfying the customer, and I'm not sure we're sensitive to timeliness. So I would say that all four of those components are quite unlike what the hospital system and medical staff have seen as their role. That's my own assessment.

Dr. Bernard Badley: Since I believe there are some unrealistic expectations, I would add a qualifier that we should aim to satisfy legitimate customer expectations. Health care providers have a job to do to educate the public about what expectations are realistic. There still is a role for using a walking stick before you have your hip replaced — those sorts of things. If we were to respond to *every* demand, we would be unable to fulfil Don's requirement of operating within an affordable system.

Schurman: One of the things I've never been able to satisfy in my own mind is whether the consumer really has unrealistic expectations. I continue to get that feedback from staff within our organization, yet I continue to resist the belief that this is necessarily the case. I'm not sure I accept that the public have unrealistic expectations.

Badley: Some do. Absolutely. Some of the expectations of relatives for continued life support, for example, are totally unreasonable. People in fact come to my office and say, "My father's in intensive care and they want to turn the machines off. We want everything possible to be done." You then find out that the patient is 98 years old, blind, atherosclerotic, and had a stroke three months ago and now has pneumonia and heart failure. I regard such a demand as unrealistic.

Patricia Henderson: I think the one thing you said, Don, was "timeliness," and the one thing that we have always done in health care is implemented, acted, and the whole bit, and we didn't talk to the customer first. I know an awful lot of "pull them off the machine" kinds of people who, if they'd been asked at the time of the trauma, at the time of the accident, there is no way heroic measures would have been implemented.

I like to look at what is quality in health care more from an ethical point of view — that we're finally going to talk to the customer, not go on the egotistical trip that we were trained to do as nurses, physicians, psychologists, and physiotherapists, believing we know what's best for them. We perpetuate *our own* need. I always swear that if I were to be admitted to one of our beds and put under the geriatric assessment team — a very comprehensive assessment — I would be in long-term care from now until the day I died. They would have no trouble finding a multidisciplinary essential need for me.

But if you put it in the context of society today, all of a sudden you and I have the right to say whether we want to be treated or don't want to be treated, whether we want to die or don't want to die. This has really come flab-dab in the face of what health care has always been. *Quality* is going to be deciding to give patients what they need, if they want it, and to be able to know what the outcome to be expected is, and to be able to say upfront, "I'm sorry, if you buy this toaster from such and such a company that is much better at making tools rather than toasters, you won't get good toast in the morning. But I recommend you go and take this other company's model and you will have good toast in the morning for 20 years" — that type of thing.

We don't even know how to say, "I'm sorry, we can't do that very well." So *quality* is when we really just give people what they request for a certain outcome and don't continue to perpetuate the need for *ourselves*.

Is there a fundamental standard of health care every community must have?

Henderson: I tend to be philosophical and I take that question back to where society is at right now. And society is now concerned with everybody asserting their individual rights. We are not going to reach what the customer wants if *we* determine what the standard of health care service is for everybody and if we aren't as flexible as we expect everybody to be for us.

Dr. Donald Carlow: It raises the question of how far the whole issue of quality really does go. If we look at quality as the total application of the knowledge that we have, and translate this into programs and public policy, then ultimately quality would be far-reaching. For example, in the case of cancer, where we know that 35 per cent of cancers are caused by smoking (bladder, pancreas, and lung) there would be a public policy that prevents the sale of cigarettes. And there is also the issue of quality of life. I don't know whether your definition, in terms of responsiveness to valid customer requirements, includes quality of life.

Schurman: That would get into more of *my* response to the question "Is there a fundamental standard, a fundamental infrastructure that every community has a right to expect?" I would answer that the same way I would answer any of our internal people who would say, "You can't cut me anymore because there's a basic level of requirement for our services." And my response would be that none of us has an inalienable right to exist.

The only right we have to exist is in direct proportion to our commitment. If the health care system has a sense of what it can deliver to a community, then there should be corresponding resources. But frankly I'm not sure that we've ever articulated what value we add to the health status of the population. Nor do any of the health professionals very often give us a sense of the "value-added" that they provide to patient care. They don't have a right to exist, nor do I think *we* have a right to exist within a community, unless we have some sense of what we're committed to deliver to the community in terms of health status.

I think when we get to the issues of what sort of interventions that some of us are undertaking in cancer care at your institution and at my hospital,

and Bernie's [Badley] place — expensive interventions — in some respects, I don't think they add much value.

Carlow: When you talk about standards of health care services that every
community must have, it raises the issue of how you work with a community to determine what that standard is or what that community would
like to have. It raises the issue of accountability and how the system is
designed in relation to how you meet the accountability function or public
expectations. So it gets back to governance of health care, and the role of
governance in relation to quality and community standards — are we
properly structured?

Henderson: Wouldn't the ultimate quality for us be that we're not
needed anymore?

*What are the points in health care that we have simply not had the courage
"to put a marker down"?*

Badley: It's not just courage, although courage may be a part of it. In
the past, when resources were adequate for all of our activities, there
wasn't the need to measure the outcomes of many of the things we do.
Now, when we need to do so, we haven't the tools or appropriate techniques. So we can't answer Don's question as to what really provides true
added value. I'm struck by the fact that 20 years ago there was a study in
which half of a group of patients referred for physiotherapy had the
diathermy lamp switched on, and for the other half, the lamp wasn't
switched on. The outcome was the same in both groups. Now that was
20 years ago, but for several years thereafter, we continued to follow
our usual customs rather than being guided by the objective outcomes
of intervention.

    Now we are beginning to ask the question, "Does the result warrant the
resources that went into the process?" However, studies like these are
extraordinarily complex, expensive, and time-consuming. If you want to
assess the outcome of a common surgical procedure, you probably need
a several-year follow-up of a large group of patients in order to see whether
in fact the intervention has significantly improved the quality of life.

Schurman: I think the onus needs to be put on each and every one of us as members of the health care team to stand for something, to make a declaration about what value we add, and then test it over time.

Badley: But there hasn't been a structure or a knowledge base in place that would allow one to say, "That's a load of baloney. It shouldn't be done in this situation. It is wasting money." We are now in a position that we'd like to say that, but we don't yet have the data on which to base such a value judgement.

Schurman: There's an interesting dialogue going on in our place as we talk about reorganizing the structure, reorganizing the allocation of re- sources around the program management structure, where the doctors and perhaps nurses may be responsible for buying services — say, physio, O.T., or social services — and all those support areas are now anxious because they're obviously afraid that someone is not going to purchase their services. They don't want to go down that road because they want to protect their resources. I say to them, "If you're out in the private sector and nobody comes through your door, then you should close. So, too, in our institution." They would say, "But the buyers don't understand the value that we add." And I say, "Then you'd better devise a sufficient relationship with those people to make sure that they do see the value in your services."

Carlow: I think that one of the major barriers in TQM is fear as it relates to the role of professional groups. We frankly have been organized around the professional disciplines, and quality as perceived by these professional groups may be quite different. Major institutions are actually there to operate within the standards of the professions as opposed to the valid customer requirements.

Will TQM expose this?

Badley: I feel it will. But it's very difficult to get people to co-operate in what they perceive as a process that is detrimental to their own profession.

The dean of medicine at the University of Western Ontario has said that if you look at the literature, only 15 or 20 per cent of what we do medically has ever been proven. Comments?

Badley: Yes, I agree that only 15 or 20 per cent of what we do has been proven. However, I would suspect that perhaps another 40 per cent is effective. I have no idea about the rest.

Henderson: One of the things I'm finding in our place is, if you want to relate all this to continuous quality improvement, that I feel very good with the employees when we are doing more on an outpatient basis. Our goal is to keep people in the community as long as possible, and get them back out into the community as soon as possible — I saw this as a real threat three or four years ago.

But there are others throughout the province who are downsizing because of the almighty buck, and not with any aspect of quality or for purposes of what they're trying to achieve. It has nothing to do with increasing productivity or becoming more efficient. When you've been this long on the journey, you get a few employees who say to you, "Thanks, at least there's a purpose to all of this," whereas there are others downsizing with no logic, no sense, no sensibility to it at all.

Schurman: The private-sector people that I spend some time with talk about ruthlessly cutting out any sort of activity that isn't value-added. That's a mentality that we probably need to apply in health care. The trouble is that it's much easier for them to make the determination than us. For example, if you are an automobile dealer where you are actually delivering the car, it is easier to go to the consumer and find out what it is they like and what it is they don't think they need, and then to cut it out. *Our* consumers still have a difficult time assessing what is value-added and what isn't, and of course, we as health professionals don't assist the public a lot to get access to that sort of knowledge. They don't know whether or not five X-rays are better than two.

Carlow: We must consider this whole TQM concept, how it's going to affect us if we're truly responding to the needs of customers. What we're going to try to do as organizations and as communities is really respond to the needs of patients in continuity across the system. This is one of the things we haven't done very well. We all function within our castles and provide that episodic element, but if we really believe in TQM, what will we do as leaders to ensure a local or community-based system that provides for responsive, seamless service delivery?

It's probably well stated in the philosophy and the statements of ethics of the American College of Health Care Executives — a statement that refers to the obligations of those who lead organizations to participate in the broader system.

Should we be adding a third word after "wants" and "needs"? Has this "needs of the community" concept really thrown us?

Schurman: I'm not sure if you need another word to substitute for "wants" or "needs." What we need is a clear articulation of some goals, of some health status indicator goals — which is so horribly done in our country. And when we tried to do it recently in Edmonton, it became so "airy-fairy," so imprecise. Yet I've seen some good work being done. I think it was New Zealand that a few years ago articulated its health goals. I believe if you can articulate some clearer health goals, the system can address the issue of needs precisely and the role that the various providers should play.

Henderson: I think everything that happens has a leader. Why are we all caught up in this? I'm finding myself saying, in inter-hospital planning and in discussions with the medical officer of health in our community, that I'm just as much a part of our being a healthy community as you are. But all of those things take leadership and risk.

Schurman: Who does the community count on to do that?

Badley: The move now to regional health authorities and councils who truly represent the community is a step in this direction. The practical problem is that their members are, in general, relatively uneducated consumers who are unaware of many of the complexities of health care. They are now going to set those goals and priorities and will distribute the available resources. That's a very nice theory but very scary in practice. Nevertheless, that's certainly the way things are going in several parts of the country. I applaud the theory, but I'm terrified of the potential results.

Henderson: Why can't *you* do it, Don?

Schurman: I don't think the biggest hospital in the city would be allowed the leadership role to try to articulate all this. It's too self-serving.

What is it that people are asking for by this involvement? The politicians or the community — what are they really after?

Badley: I think it's a reaction to the paternalistic face of medicine that's been present for many centuries. I can say, as a member of the medical profession, that we have seen ourselves as the high priests; we have always told you what's good for you. You have a sickness; I have a menu of cures; you will fit into one of them. That's the traditional thing. But people are now saying, "We really haven't been given sufficient information and proven facts to make informed choices."

This is an appropriate reaction to paternalistic provider attitude. However, it's equally wrong, I think, to swing over entirely to the other side and say that the consumer now sets the entire stage. You really need someone in the middle.

Henderson: It always blows my mind that the lady where I buy my clothes has the guts to tell me, "That looks terrible on you, Pat," and wouldn't sell me something that looked terrible on me. But I walk into my doctor's office and my doctor says to me, "Well now, try this, Pat. Now I'm not so sure it's going to work. Come back in six days if you're not feeling well." But the person in the dress shop, she won't let me walk out of that store with something she doesn't think is right.

Badley: Let me pick up on that, because one of the other consumer groups we have to deal with is our physicians. In fact, saying to a patient: "Try this for six days, see if it helps, come back if it doesn't," may be the most cost-effective form of therapy.

Dr. Brent James [of Intermountain Healthcare Inc. in Utah] divides physicians into "optimalists" and "maximalists." The tradition, which has been clothed with the misnomer of "academic" medicine, has been to do every conceivable test to prove things to the hilt before we do anything. This is a maximalist way of doing things, and is a reflection of traditional medical educational culture.

For example, I'm a gastroenterologist and I want to get a radiological test done. Radiologists now have so many different modalities that they may do an initial study, and then say "Now you need a CT scan, followed by an isotope study and, perhaps, an MRI." They do so to nail the problem down to the most precise degree they can by radiological means. That's the objective of their discipline.

My objective as a clinician is quite different. I have to make an operational decision and I need to ask: "What's the least amount of information that I require to make that decision?"

The question may be, "Is it important that I refer him to a surgeon now or is it safe for me to put him on medication for several days and see if it makes things better?" Often the initial test is all that is needed to allow me to make that choice.

The additional information might be interesting but is not critical in making the decision. The "optimalist" point of view seeks the least amount of information needed to make a management decision. The two approaches have very different cost implications.

Who leads us out of this?

Schurman: I think we've already begun to answer that. You know it can't be completely the consumers themselves because I think there are issues which require the insights of professionals. So there presumably has to be some sort of a dialogue between the health professions and the community.

Carlow: As we restructure the way we deliver care, we should consider the scope of program management. Maybe the way we link with the community is not only broadly-based, but related to specific program areas.

One of the issues we're dealing with right now as an organization, and I think it's a national issue, is breast cancer research. Who decides where the resources go in breast cancer research? We're an organization that has six major breast cancer research programs and we're very proud of them, and they cover all the important areas. But who makes those decisions? The National Cancer Institute, the Medical Research Council, National Institutes of Health. These organizations have little to do directly with any group of people who have the disease. We need to consult with organizations that deal with the patients, such as the Canadian Breast Cancer Foundation, in order to determine the priorities.

Schurman: That's the issue. We're used to provider dominance and maybe we've organized the system to meet our needs as administrators and doctors. We've organized the research structure to meet the needs of the research community.

Is this concern with community input one way of expressing the whole CQI agenda? We've never really asked our consumers. We've never really understood that part of the system.

Badley: It's true, we haven't used these measures for two reasons. If we *knew* what people really wanted, we would have been able to make better decisions. We have not had the answers to either of these questions, but CQI does, in fact, address them. It says, "Let's ask the consumer," and then "Let's identify the measures" that are needed to answer some of these questions relating to the effectiveness of what we do.

Schurman: I wonder if CQI is driving us or if CQI is being driven by something else. I could argue, I think, that there's a worldwide shift toward democratization. You can see it in Eastern Europe, but you can also see it in our organizations, in the staff who are demanding some say, and in consumers, whether it's with respect to cars or health care. I might argue that the sweep toward democratization drives some different approaches to management.

Badley: CQI is a response, one of the first *logical* responses.

What is it that is really making us decide in the direction of total quality management? Is it "I can improve the process" or something else more fundamental? Secondly, are we really leading the health care system out of its morass, or do we just want to be on the leading edge of public relations or the leading edge of our communities?

Badley: The driving force to me is the survival of my institution, not in the competitive sense of the U.S., but in the desire to continue to provide those things we have an obligation to provide. Our funding is decreasing. We have to reduce or eliminate some of the things we currently do, and if we don't make the decisions more intelligently, we'll end up with illogical across-the-board cuts that run the danger of removing some of the things that are good for our patients, as well as some things that aren't. Right now I'm not quite sure which are all the "good ones" and which are all the "bad ones."

Sister Mary Jean Ryan: I would just offer one thing at this point because I think there's an aspect of this that the U.S. systems are in the process of dealing with. We're beginning to look at some fairly serious erosion of our bottom line. That's fortunately somewhat new to us. In the last seven years we've had some fairly successful years. One of the immediate things that everybody races to do, of course, is lay off staff. That's a fairly significant way to cut some expenses. The notion of cutting is something that we've been very reluctant to do, simply because if you cut services, it's going to take you 10 years to bring those back and you can have some very good services going on. The other thing we've come to realize is that there are some immediate things that you can do. Everything that you do now will have an impact at some time not too far into the future that could be far worse than what we're currently experiencing. Frankly, we've looked at reductions in labour force as the easiest way out of things. It's the easiest way for a manager to deal with it, but it's also the worst.

Carlow: Someone asked why we're doing this. Is it relative to customers or to the imperatives that are out there? Is it also that we all want to be the best leaders that we can possibly be, and that we'll do anything that is appropriate or that is state-of-the-art leadership in order to get there? That's why some of us are doing it. We just want to be good leaders.

That drives *me*, I must tell you. I think I'm developing as a leader and I want to know what leadership is, and I read a great deal about it. I want to do it. So I'm trying to do it. And I think *that* drives some of us.

Also, the organization — we all want to be proud of our organizations. We want to create workplaces where people are happy, motivated, involved, and proud. This motivates me to do this. I really want to see this environment in our organization.

Henderson: I see it as a vehicle for the future. Part of it is. I heard everybody here discussing the community and TQM. We have to take ownership that *we* have broken down all those links, whether it be with the public health unit or with another hospital, or perhaps you're perceived as the largest hospital. We're part of that and we have to take ownership of it — and we have some peace bridges to build.

It's hard to build a peace bridge with somebody else if you haven't got your own act together, if you're all of a sudden in the mud and you're not sure you're going to be able to come up for the next breath or whether you're just going to have to close another 50 beds. I see this [TQM] as a way for our staff. I want to sit down and talk with the physiotherapists and say, "What can we do together, and it's probably going to mean that we might have three less physiotherapists, but together with one bit of equipment we can serve this community." You have to get your own act together. Your own staff have to feel involved. They have to trust that whatever you are doing is for the best. If you don't do this type of thing in your own organization, you won't be successful in sitting down with the rest of the community to make it happen.

I see TQM as a phenomenal vehicle for the preferred future. Yes, for survival, but it's a vehicle that's going to get us to a preferred future.

Schurman: I strongly believe in what Don [Carlow] articulated, that it's a vehicle to design a much better workplace which will be good for customers and the staff. But I also have a deep concern about our health care system, and I think this is a vehicle to help maintain that system.

I believe that our system is one of the icons of Canada. It's one of the things that creates a distinction between ourselves in Canada and our friends to the south in the U.S. I suggest that you can't separate our health care system from the notion of what it means to be a Canadian. Now maybe I'm conceptualizing at too high a level, but I feel quite strongly about it. If you ask people on the street, "What are some of the real differences between us and people in the States?", one of the first things they'll talk about is the health care system. They'll talk about the Canadian commitment to peacekeeping, as well, but I think the health care system will be one of the distinctions they make. So I think it's both — it's maintaining the system that we're proud of as Canadians and building better workplaces.

Do you mean the system or the care that we provide?

Schurman: There's a difference. In a comparison of the level of satisfaction with our system to the U.S. system, Canadians, depending on the research project study selected, rated their level of satisfaction with our system as high as 80 per cent, while the Americans rated their level of satisfaction with their system as low as 10 or 20 per cent. But when you ask an individual American who has access to the system about their level of satisfaction with their most recent hospitalization, and when you ask that same question of a Canadian, they will score better in the U.S.

So I speak about improving the system because, from a population point of view, that's a better question than one's individual experience. We shouldn't ignore the fact, however, that some individual people accessing the system are not content with the system, and we should use the tools and techniques of TQM to improve the individual level of satisfaction as well.

Can you describe two or three things that you see in front of you as leaders in this CQI transformation — in developing yourselves, developing your organization, in being part of this health care system?

Badley: One of the major obstacles to achieving a more effective system is the current method of funding professional services. When people are paid for doing more — fee for service — it's very difficult to change from the maximalist to the optimalist view. However, the obstacle is not just money. It includes professional status and autonomy. All the players in the system need to develop common goals, and that's a process that is beginning but that isn't going to happen quickly.

Carlow: As we face the facts of life every day, for example, we're faced with a zero per cent environment, an operating plan development process that must involve the community, and be approved by the district health council. How do we continue to motivate and interest people in CQI when they are faced with all of these other things? These days there is a very, very long agenda of organizational change.

I worry, too, that as an organization with 1,500 people and with 150 involved in CQI, that we've got a long way to go. I worry about that, and I guess I really would like to move faster, but I know that's wrong.

That's actually what keeps me going. I think about this as long-term, and what we're really doing is transforming the organization over a period of five to seven years. When I think about that, I relax, and I don't worry quite so much. I don't worry so much about the facts of life that we face every day.

I think about the medical staff and their commitment and how to effectively involve them. I really believe that fundamentally their culture is very compatible with CQI in terms of quantitative methods and data-driven processes. So far I've been pleased to see people in our organization responding very positively to it and saying, "Finally administration has arrived and now they're going to manage and lead based upon facts instead of upon subjective opinion." We can talk about CQI projects in housekeeping and a variety of support departments, but really the business we're in is providing clinical services to patients. So another obstacle, another challenge for us, is that of organizational design or redesign in relation to the product, and how we can focus that on patients.

Schurman: I have a significant concern about our capability as individual contributors in the health care system to really make this work. In Japan, virtually all of their successful companies have been applying this approach for 30 or 40 years. But how many had to die? Survival of the fittest may exist so that now they have a network of industries within their country that are extremely proficient. The Germans do it in a different way. The Japanese are not, however, applying this approach to their health care system. In North America, while we all talk about some great successes in the U.S. and Canada, from Motorola to General Electric to a few others, there are still relatively few who have mastered this. And while I'm not familiar with everything taking place in the United States, I haven't seen very many examples of clear, systemic sorts of break-throughs in the way an entire organization works.

I see remarkable incidences of improvement in our institution and in many other institutions, but fundamental transformation I haven't seen. Knowing about all of the issues that have been raised — alignment, reward and recognition, organization structure, and recognizing the complexity of health care — I am concerned about whether or not we're able to get the job done even though the approach makes sense and it should work. I'm convinced the script has not been written.

Finally, I am concerned that if we can't achieve improvements, the staff may give up on us as leaders, and then I think we've really lost it.

Henderson: My vision is that there's going to be fewer of us. Common sense is going to prevail pretty soon, that you don't downsize here a bit, and downsize a bit here, and downsize a bit here. I am very, very determined — this is going to sound egotistical — that my leadership and my willingness to learn, hour by hour, day by day, better ways to do things, and to lead staff, that I'm going to be one of the few left.

There are going to be fewer health institutions, and the best are going to survive. I want to be part of the best. I don't worry about it. I know that's the way it's going to be, and I don't worry whether physicians are fee-for-service or not, because by the time we'll have arrived at that point, physicians are also going to redefine their role and their relationship with us. I just know that's the way it's going to be. *I* may not be there, but our organization will be there.

I don't understand your second concern. We must be willing to look around. Do you know that the Shouldice Hospital sitting right here in Toronto is one of the best in the world for meeting the needs of the customer, and doing so much and giving the lowest cost? You can go to Greater Victoria if you're worried about how you communicate with your community and see a great leader in Ken Fyke and what he did, and here sits Sister Mary Jean Ryan, and I've been several places. We've got examples.

Schurman: We've got examples and I'm an optimist. I considered leaving the health care system until I became aware of this approach, but I still haven't seen breakthrough levels of performance. I have a hunch that we're going to see something significant in two to three years. We've got wonderful individual success stories throughout the University of Alberta Hospitals, and we should try to understand why it works in a few areas. You don't have to go to Victoria or to Shouldice because you can see it within your own institutions, and yet to see it permeate the whole organization is another question.

Henderson: Do you know I talk about your successes all the time? I stand up and I say, "Do you know University of Alberta Hospitals reduced their grievances by 600 per cent?"

Badley: There is a difference in degree of complexity between Motorola and a hospital. Motorola has a single product.

Schurman: I am damn sure that out of our $260 million budget, there's probably $75 to $80 million that should be dropping out of that budget without any compromise to the quality of care. My point is I'm not sure if we've invented the processes, the systems, the necessary alignment to get it done. That doesn't mean we're not going to do it — I'm absolutely prepared to make that commitment. In fact, I've gone out in the organization and said, "I request commitment to reducing costs by 30 per cent over three years providing the same range of services at the current volumes. And that we will create together the tools."

Carlow: But aren't we expecting too much too soon? I know we're nibbling at the edges. Yes, there have been some breakthroughs and you've given some examples, Pat, but really I think our organizations have to understand, and hopefully they will, that if they really *know* CQI, it is going to take a long time. As we continue to work within our institutions and across institutions, and with the community, the breakthroughs will come, but it's going to be a few years down the road before a significant number of those count.

Our role as leaders is, I think, to be patient, to be consistent and to be persistent. Play this game like Ben Hogan played golf. The guy never gave up. He never stopped going to the practice fairway and he became the best, and I think that's really what it takes.

Henderson: We must also be willing to share. We can't wait for each one of us to keep reinventing the wheel. All those story boards up [at the conference] — we've never shared the intricacies of how we accomplished this. If you've got it all solved on hip replacements, why aren't we doing hip replacements like that across Canada?

Badley: Again, I can't over-stress the complexity of modern health care. I started to count how many different "small businesses" there are in our hospital and I quit. There may be about 400. How do you get all 400 to progress at the same rate? It's impossible.

We have to produce a climate in which each of those 400 groups feels uncomfortable if it's not moving toward mutually accepted vision of the future, and we need to build in a reward-and-recognition system that encourages them in their efforts.

But there have always been examples of empowerment. For example, many intensive-care units have functioned for years as teams in which the nurses, technologists, and physicians are all vital players in making group decisions.

I think one of the big changes is in the physicians who now recognize they must be part of the solution of institutional problems. For decades there has been a sense of antagonism between physicians and administrators. That's now beginning to change and the "we" and "they" attitude is rapidly breaking down. That's a major paradigm shift.

Philip Hassen: The underlying point is that we need to break it down to its pieces and enable the pieces to occur, because *we're* not going to do it. We are going to lead but we're not going to *do* it. *They're* going to do it. We've got to give staff the stimulation to do it. That theme is clearly there among the four of you. The question of leadership is fundamental, and on the point of transformation, it's my view that there's going to be some kind of inversion or conversion. Who knows what it's going to look like, but it's going to be different.

Do you believe that the organizational cultures of entire hospitals will change in a positive direction?

Schurman: Juran suggests that self-directed work teams may be the predominant form of organization in the future. I think we will see a fundamental change in the nature of management. There will be fewer managers. I think we'll see the system change as Pat has outlined. Hospitals as we know them will be remarkably different. There will be fewer of us. We are quickly coming to grips with the issue of alignment of medical staff within institutions, and the problems that Bernard raised, I think, are going to be gone. I think there's the political will, there's the public will, and there's even a will within the professions to get this monkey (cost increases and a declining health care system) off their back. So I believe we will see realignment take place with entire institutional cultures shifting.

Henderson: What always amazes me is that we have had self-directed work teams in hospitals for the 30 years that I've been there. The administrator left on Friday, and staff handled emergencies and everything else very beautifully. We kept the hospital going until the leader got back on Monday morning. And yet it's taken somebody all this time to convince me about self-directed work teams.

Schurman: I don't believe your assessment is necessarily accurate. When I first joined the University Hospital, vice-presidents were on call. We got called to open up another bed. We got called about what to do with certain patient concerns. We got called about everything. So it's not true that the staff were empowered and in control.

Badley: But the examples were there. The intensive-care unit with cross-functional teams, the nurses have been empowered, there have been group decisions — we've had perfect examples.

Henderson: And highly efficient. You get out of a coronary intensive-care unit much faster than you get out of a medical bed these days.

Carlow: I think we have some very good examples of customer-focused care in our system — not acute-care hospitals — but long-term care facilities. I think probably, in many respects, they've led the way in being much more customer-focused and responsive to the needs of the elderly and building them into the system of care, and designing the facilities after consultation with these people to create an appropriate environment. We went through some of this in developing geriatric programs on the West Coast a number of years ago. Yet it's just sinking into acute care.

Badley: I think one of the big changes we're going to see is in the physicians who now recognize that they've got to be part of the solution and not the entire problem. There has been for decades that antagonism between them and us. You know, "We do the work around here and you administrators screw us up and don't provide us with enough resources." I've been saying that for 30 years. I think that's beginning to change and the "we" and "them" is rapidly breaking down. That's a major paradigm shift.

Carlow: I agree with that, and I think we're going to see a fundamental restructuring that's related to the way we manage resources, deliver care, manage quality through multi- or interdisciplinary teams relative to clinical products involving physicians, and through a horizontal stream, linking the community through a broad-based array of services. I think that's what we're going to see.

Schurman: We're talking mainly from the provider point of view about some of the changes. I think things are going to change from the patient's point of view within hospitals. I think we're going to move from the notion of informed consent, which I'm beginning to find offensive, to empowered choice. It would be nice to develop a presentation on that because, as I analyse more closely this notion of informed consent, I find it objectionable. It means that we intimidate the patient into some sort of consent so that the provider can intervene in his or her preferred way.

What needs to be in place in hospitals and communities to create the seamless health care system of the future — from community to hospital and back to community?

Carlow: Well, I think that's going to vary depending upon what issue, product, or program you're really talking about. If you're talking about testicular cancer or talking about prostatic cancer or talking about breast cancer, or talking about leukemia, or whatever it might be — it might be quite different. The community resources might be quite different. The volunteer agencies might be quite different, et cetera, et cetera. I think it's going to have to be tailored to the specific requirements of that particular issue. I don't think there's any standard formula.

Schurman: It will be a natural evolution. If we begin to appreciate that within institutions everything happens as a process that cuts across the organization, you can then view the patient being admitted to the hospital, going through a treatment, and being discharged as a process. It doesn't seem difficult then to define the process and to begin discussion throughout the system in an attempt to design a "seamless" process from the customer's point of view.

What is required, however, is sufficient time to have a critical mass of health care providers in a community commit to this approach so the conversations are possible.

Badley: I think you're going to have to demonstrate effectiveness within your own institution before you can expect a buy-in from other institutions. They want to be part of a success story. They currently have their own individual autonomy, and they're not likely to surrender it willingly unless they can see it's for a better process.

To close, will you name one thing you are proud of right now as a leader, as a change agent, as a CEO, in the context of this agenda of transformation through total quality management?

Schurman: I can't point to any specific event. I can only speak to the relationships among staff. For example, I would point to environmental services and housekeeping staff. Due to the different management approach TQM brings about, there is a rapport between staff and senior management that hasn't been seen before. The culture in the organization, the mood of the organization, is changing and that is the one thing I am most proud of.

Badley: I agree. Nurses who've been away raising kids for two or three years will come down to my office and say, "This place is different." You can't put numbers on that. I've been away from my hospital for two weeks now and I haven't had a phone call. *That* wouldn't have happened three or four years ago. they're little things, but they represent a significant change in the culture of our organization.

Carlow: Well, I could tell you it's getting a $235 million capital project approved in extremely difficult times and through an extremely difficult and political process with the city of Toronto and the government of Ontario. But it's not really been that. I could also say it's total corporate restructuring in a fairly short period of time, the recruiting of good people, and developing a good organization. But really what it is, I think, is moving from an organization which about four years ago was very, very controlling, central, and very directed with power in the hands of two people, to one that's moving out, and where people are happy to come to work. I know we have a long way to go, but that transformation is occurring. I worry about it a lot, but it is happening and I feel better about that than the three-storey hole that's in the ground right now on University Avenue.

Henderson: I think I'm proudest, right now at this moment, because I can literally say that TQM has been embodied in the total organization. And we successfully did it with a board of directors who are ready to start benchmarking in quality with another hospital. We successfully did it with the volunteers, and when you get 500 to 600 volunteers embodying it, you've all of a sudden reached out into your community, because it is now more than your staff. And we successfully were able to do it with the residents and family council. It really is different when you start to respond to family and patient complaints with possible good solutions and options — that's accountability with feedback. That's what I'm proudest of. Now, tomorrow it might be something else, but right at this moment, that's what I'm proudest of.

Sister Mary Jean: I guess all of the above, because we're dealing with 22 facilities. But the stories are very much as you've told them. I think that actually I could probably go home now, because you've all referenced certain parts of the presentation I'm going to give later today. I think it's the attitudinal changes. You know, I have what we call hands-on healers in our system, that is, people who have no management responsibility, who come to me and say, "Thank you very much for CQI." It says to me that there are some really significant things happening. I don't expect to see us achieve the measure of things that I would like to achieve. I'm not going to live that long. But I am going to be able to say that we've put in place the structures that are necessary to achieve that, because we also then have 4,000 physicians and 15,000 employees who are, I think, eager for this. Those that aren't will have to find jobs someplace else.

Hassen: To wrap this dialogue up, first, I'm proud, like you, that we're beginning to get feedback *even* from physicians, if I may say so, because they suddenly are beginning to realize that this is an important solution for all of us. From the staff person who writes me a little note saying, "I didn't realize what this was going to mean to me but I now understand it," or from a staff person who has just been trained and says, "I now have hope" — it's all those things that begin to embody this cultural change. I don't think we're there. We're culturally shifting. I am nervous — I work in a Catholic hospital and every time I tell the Sisters the culture is changing, I sense they get nervous about the values possibly changing. The reality is that the values are what make us the strongest. We're very fortunate that what we're doing aligns well with the values. That's the easy part.

Second, I am proud of the leadership that I see around this room right now. I'm pleased to be part of what you people are a part of and what you're doing, because this is what's going to make the difference. This is what's going to lead us out of our current difficulties. We'll see other things that will dream for us or with us, but I think we've got to drive ahead, as was said, in a way that allows us to continue this journey, because it's very, very important to our society — to Canadian society as a whole — I think also to our staff and to the people we serve.

Participants

DONALD SCHURMAN is president and CEO of Edmonton's 1,200-bed University of Alberta Hospitals, where some 120 teams have participated in TQM since 1989.

DR. BERNARD BADLEY is president and CEO of Victoria General Hospital in Halifax, Nova Scotia. This 800-bed tertiary care facility began its TQM initiative in 1990.

PATRICIA HENDERSON is executive director and CEO of the Freeport Hospital Health Care Village in Kitchener, Ontario, a unique chronic care and rehabilitation facility that began TQM two years ago.

DR. DONALD CARLOW is president and CEO of the Ontario Cancer Institute/Princess Margaret Hospital, a facility in Toronto that serves 150,000 patients annually and began TQM in 1991.

SISTER MARY JEAN RYAN is president and CEO of the 4,000-bed SSM (Sisters of St. Mary) Health Care System based in St. Louis, Missouri, which implemented TQM in 1989 at all of its 22 sites.

9

What Does the Future Hold?

The important thing is not to stop questioning. Curiosity has its own reason for existing. One cannot help but be in awe when he contemplates the mysteries of eternity, of life, of the marvellous structure of reality. It is enough if one tries merely to comprehend a little of this mystery every day — never lose a holy curiosity.

— ALBERT EINSTEIN

The world is now in a time of profound turmoil. The systems of the past — political, economic, and social — are in flux. The more optimistic among political and economic analysts speak of this global instability, with its fallout pressures on employment, productivity and social systems, as an "economic restructuring" or "organizational destructuring" that will eventually bottom out and then begin a recovery. The more pessimistic refer to it as a "breakdown" or "falling apart" of the social order and believe that much of the economic and social damage may be irreversible.

Whatever we choose to call what is happening to us both locally and globally, it *is* increasingly a time of social and organizational chaos. If we have been reading newspaper articles or watching TV features on the recession, the numerous business closures, the strife of war-torn countries, the creation of new nations, and starvation in Third-World countries, or have even just talked to family members, colleagues, or neighbours who have suffered job layoffs or bankruptcies, we are struck by the awareness that there is no stability virtually anywhere on earth.

All systems — government, education, legal, social welfare, and health care — are under severe external and internal pressure for change. Many are trying to conceptualize the change but to date few have created demonstrable changes, partly because they are trying to use maps in uncharted territory. This would be like asking Christopher Columbus what map he used to get to his destination. More intuitive, high-risk oriented leadership is necessary to make non-linear leaps in thinking in order to find new solutions for tomorrow. Compasses, signals, and signposts are needed instead of well laid-out maps.

For most of these societal institutions, the time of plenty is no more. A much more foreboding task is at hand. Health care systems will be as susceptible to these forces of destructuring as any other organized system in our society, organizational analyst Leland Kaiser told participants at a San Francisco health care conference in fall 1992.

Kaiser places the destructuring of societal institutions within the context of a dying paradigm. The organizational and conceptual categories we have grown up with over the past few generations no longer serve us. Even the way we frame our questions — Is this a move to the political right or the left? Is this a redistribution of power or a retrenchment of power? — does not lead us to enlightening answers because the questions themselves are of the old paradigm. Much of what is happening today defies categories. We cannot deal with the new by using old mental models or worn-out definitions and methodologies. We cannot at this point even predict with any accuracy what the new will be.

For health care institutions faced with hard new realities and considerable confusion as to what to do about them, two paths become evident. They can descend further into an abyss and fight increasingly losing battles to deliver a high standard of health care. Or they can turn the time of chaos into a time of transformation and create health care institutions that *will* work in the emerging new world. While this book has dealt primarily with the story of only one hospital — St. Joseph's Health Centre — which is in the process of re-creating itself to meet the health care needs of the future, I believe the imperative for such change in health care is global, not just local.

THE NEED FOR NEW STRATEGIES IS SHARED WORLDWIDE
A report on the health care industry, published in early 1992 as part of the International Quality Study (IQS), looked at health care quality management practices in four countries — Canada, the U.S., Germany, and

Japan. "Findings indicate that a global concern for quality patient care has brought a convergence of practices in several areas," the report states. "For example, substantial numbers of hospitals in all four countries are planning to increasingly use technology to satisfy patients, referring physicians, and other customers, and to improve service delivery. Additionally, participants in Canada, Germany, Japan, and the United States indicate they plan to apply more stringent quality criteria to suppliers, provide more cross-training to employees, and continue to integrate various elements of the patient-care delivery process, particularly the nursing function.

"In some areas of human resource practices and use of quality tools, a distinct North American hospital quality improvement approach is emerging. Other findings indicate that hospitals in all four countries have not yet fully applied classical quality management principles."[1]

In other words, there is still a long way to go. Even Japan, the undisputed world leader in industrial and corporate quality, has in terms of health care, according the IQS report, tended to emphasize quality outcomes but has not yet paid a lot of attention to the area of patient satisfaction. And, similar to Germany, Japan's hospitals are geared to a "top down" decision-making process in which boards of directors and physicians are responsible for the development and clinical management of most new services. And in much of North America, under the old paradigm, it is senior management that plays this decision-making role. "Hospitals in all four nations have yet to address customer expectations in a systematic way," the report observes.[2]

The report details some of the societal, economic, and demographic forces driving each of the four nations increasingly toward making choices that will favour strategies of continuous quality improvement. In Canada, it is recessionary pressure combined with constraints on public spending. For Canadian hospitals, issues of continued access to health care are in the foreground, particularly concerns with health care rationing and patient waiting lists.

In Germany, the dominant role of the physician and the tight regulatory government control of hospitals has meant that continuous quality improvement is not, as yet, often raised as a specific issue. But the German health care system faces some significant challenges over the next few years, in particular the need to integrate 16 million citizens from what was formerly East Germany into Germany's national health insurance.

The IQS report notes another interesting development in Europe arising from efforts to create a unified European Community. This is "the emergence of what some have called the 'medical tourist' — an individual who seeks treatment in other countries if dissatisfied with that available at home. In the future, questions of access for these individuals — and the need to address the expectations of such a 'pan-European customer' on the macro level — may become issues for all hospitals across that continent."3

An enormous quality-related health care issue in Japan is that the country's population is aging faster than that of any other industrialized nation, a demographic reality Japanese hospitals, which normally provide both acute and long-term care must face. The Japanese have the greatest length — 52 days — of average hospital stay of all four countries in the study, reflecting the fact that their hospitals provide services to elderly patients who, in the West, are usually given care in nursing homes or other long-term care facilities.

While the Japanese have access to high-quality care at almost half the cost of care in the United States, the report observes that Japanese hospitals are under increasing pressure from government, businesses, and individuals to implement better cost controls.

Access to care is a major area of concern for the U.S., with almost 37 million people not covered by health insurance. The U.S. is also beleaguered by rapidly escalating health care costs — the highest in the world — coupled with a growing insistence on cost-containment efforts from both public and private payors. "The slim operating margins of U.S. hospitals require an organization-wide approach to driving costs out of systems and increasing efficiencies," the IQS report says. "Not surprisingly, CQI tools that simplify and improve cross-functional business processes are particularly attractive to U.S. hospitals."4

The IQS evaluated hospitals in only four countries, but many of the points made in the report have worldwide relevance. No country anywhere today has unlimited resources for health care or any other social program. Access, effectiveness, efficiency, and cost restraints are issues for all. Even though many European countries spend less than North America on health care in general, and manage to better contain the costs of treating their elderly patients in particular, the aging of European and North American populations will have a significant impact on health systems in future.

"Likewise," suggests the IQS report, "continuing advances in technology and medical treatment carry increasingly expensive price tags in all nations. Managing those costs — as well as managing quality — will continue to be mandates for all hospital leaders."5

In future, then, if hospitals are to evolve into insitutions of total quality, their decision-makers will need to extend their quest for innovation, improved treatment procedures, and organizational change beyond their walls to the health care experiences and practices in other parts of the world.

TOTAL QUALITY CANADIAN- AND AMERICAN-STYLE

All industrialized nations with publicly funded health care systems spend considerable resources on health care. Canada, Sweden, Germany, Denmark, France, New Zealand, and numerous other developed countries have in common the struggle to maintain universal accessibility to their health care systems while controlling escalating costs. But in Canada the dilemma is particularly troublesome. Canada has the most expensive health care system of all countries that publicly fund health care; it sits on the border, and thus nearer the influence of, the one powerful nation whose health care system is primarily funded through private insurance. Health care in the United States is paid for by a mix of employer-purchased insurance coverage, private insurance plans, and such government programs as Medicare and Medicaid, targeted primarily — many also say ineffectively — at the poor and elderly.

"Indeed, the United States is the only one of the 24 nations belonging to the Organization for Economic Co-operation and Development (OECD) where public funding accounts for less than 50 per cent of the nation's total health spending," writes Leslie Greenwald in a recent issue of *Health Management Quarterly*.6

Thirty-seven million Americans have no health coverage at all, a state of affairs an increasing number of critical American thinkers say should no longer be tolerated. Leland Kaiser, for example, suggests the lack of universal access to health care in the U.S. is immoral. Yet ironically, the U.S. spends a larger proportion of its wealth on health care than any other country — an estimated 14 per cent of GNP for 1992 whereas, to quote the July 1992 issue of *Consumer Reports* magazine, "not a single developed country other than the U.S. devotes more than 10 per cent of its gross national product to health care."7

Some analysts believe that Canada's close proximity to the U.S. plays a role in driving Canadian health care costs up. While Canadians adhere to the principles of universally accessible health care shared by most European nations, many aspects of our lifestyle, economics, and political thinking are influenced by American market-driven forces rather than by the social democratic flavour of much of Europe. "It is interesting to note that the two countries that have the highest health-spending-to-GDP ratios (Canada and the United States) also place the greatest reliance on fee-for-service reimbursement," observes Greenwald.[8]

Not surprisingly, since the mid-1980s, a number of U.S. hospitals have taken the lead in the attempt to implement total quality management as a competitive strategy to keep them viable in the U.S. health care marketplace. When I began in 1989 to explore the possibilities of total quality management in a Canadian health care setting, virtually all the information and existing examples of total quality management in action were from the U.S. For American health administrators, and for increasingly cost-vigilant insurance providers, the potential of total quality management to identify and recapture wasted resources has been one of its greatest drawing cards. And for some, the marketing strategy has been even more fundamental.

The July 1992 *Consumer Reports*, in a series of in-depth articles on the costs of the health system, estimates that of the $817 billion spent on U.S. health care in 1992, $200 billion was wasted on "overpriced, useless, even harmful treatments, and on a bloated bureaucracy."[9] However, such massive spending on health care has not resulted in better overall health outcomes. In fact, the U.S. fares rather badly on several key public health indicators. Of the 24 OECD countries, the U.S. ranks twenty-first in its infant mortality rate, seventeenth in male life expectancy, and sixteenth in female life expectancy.

"We [Americans] are no healthier than the citizens of comparable developed countries that spend half what we do and provide health care for everybody. In fact, by important measures such as life expectancy and infant mortality, we are far down the list," states *Consumer Reports*.[10] The writer then tackles the central issue that has led many hospitals to explore total quality management.

"No matter what corner of the health-care system is examined — hospital costs, clinical procedures, administrative expenses — at least 20 per cent seems to represent waste or inefficiency. If the system could be redesigned to get rid of this excess, it could, in effect, provide 20 per cent more necessary service without costing any more than it does now.

"Granted, devising a totally efficient system would be difficult, if not impossible, to accomplish. However, there is easily more than enough excess spending in our current system to take care of the roughly 14 per cent of the population who are not currently under any public or private insurance plan."[11]

It would be unfair to imply that total quality management in American hospitals, particularly in institutions that have shown strong leadership in the quality movement, such as the University of Michigan Hospitals or Intermountain Health Care Inc., is driven solely by concerns for profits or by the need to attract holders of good insurance-coverage policies.

There is a growing sense of urgency among many U.S. health care decision-makers, as well as among much of the American public, of the need to restructure the health system in the direction of greater accessibility. One 1990 survey of public attitudes toward health care involving ten countries, found that 60 per cent of American respondents thought their health system needed fundamental changes, and 29 per cent thought it should be completely rebuilt. In Canada, by comparison, only 38 per cent said the system needed fundamental changes, and just five per cent wanted the system rebuilt. One interesting aspect of this study, however, was that while U.S. respondents were the most dissatisfied with their health system, a good portion (one-third to one-half) of respondents of all the other countries in the survey (which included Canada, the Netherlands, Germany, France, Australia, Sweden, Japan, the United Kingdom, and Italy) also wanted some fundamental changes.[12]

Berwick in *Curing Health Care* acknowledges the American health system's many strengths, particularly in the advances in technological and medical treatment made possible by research and development, but he goes on to observe that in many ways "it is the worst of times for American health care, at least since it entered the scientific era of twentieth-century practice. Almost no one is happy with the health care system. It costs too much; it excludes too many; it fails too often; and it knows too little about its own effectiveness."[13]

Another strong advocate of total quality management is Sister Mary Jean Ryan, the president and CEO of the SSM Health Care System, headquartered in St. Louis, Missouri, and involving over 4,000 hospital beds and 15,500 staff. During the October 1992 "Owning the Future" conference in Toronto, she said that strategies of continuous quality improvement have the potential to call forth the innovative and creative abilities of health care administrators and health care professionals to solve some of the gravest U.S. health care system problems — specifically the lack of access, the runaway costs, and gaps in medical knowledge concerning which treatments achieve the most effective outcomes. Speaking of the quality journey as a process of entering into an open space that begins as despair and ends as hope, she challenged participants from both sides of the border to make health care the standard for, not just the equal of, industry excellence. "We have the power to begin health care again," she said.

Also being heard increasingly in the debate are the voices of the American people themselves. An influential factor in sweeping the Democrats into power in the November 1992 election was Bill Clinton's promise to make the creation of an equitable health care system a top priority. This will be a formidable task, for it will involve far more than implementing total quality management strategies, as crucial as these are for recouping the system's tremendous waste and inefficiencies. There will be powerful lobbies against reform from much of the insurance industry as well as from some vocal hospitals' and physicians' groups. There will be the problem of how to downsize the massive health care structure to the flatter, more efficient organizational model that aligns itself with total quality management while taking into account the existing excess capacity of facilities and of thousands of health care professionals.

In Canada, the process of implementing total quality management strategies will likely be less daunting. Many health care and business writers have noted that Canada, as well as other countries with universally accessible health care systems, does a better job controlling health care costs because the funding processes for health care are not as complex as those in the U.S. and tend to be more strictly regulated. It is estimated that currently 18 to 20 per cent of an American hospital's resources are used for administration. In Canada, the average is 7 to 11 per cent (at St. Joseph's, it is 7 per cent).

The complexities of dealing with an array of third-party payors — such as insurance companies and utilization-review firms — as well as government and state programs leads to much time in American hospitals being devoted to bureaucracy, paper chases, and collecting on inpatient accounts. At St. Joseph's, I spend less than five per cent of my time dealing

with the Health Centre's finances. Our accounts-receivable department
has only seven full-time staff compared to many times that amount of
accounts-receivable staff in every American health institution half the
size.

Physicians in the U.S. also must devote considerably more time to the
financial aspects of their practices. One of the misconceptions about
Canadian health care widely held by U.S. critics of the Canadian system
is that the government bureaucracy responsible for funding health care
is more complex and more interfering than the funding procedures in the
U.S. Dr. Michael Rachlis, a Toronto physician and policy consultant, is
quoted in a *Consumer Reports* article: "In the U.S. there's a myth that
Canadians have an awful government bureaucracy that tells doctors how
to practise medicine. There's much more interference from third parties
(such as insurance companies and utilization-review firms) in the U.S.
than from the government in Canada."[14]

Total quality management initiatives in Canada have also had an easier
time arousing physician interest. It is my impression that for many
American health institutions, total quality management is an extremely
hard sell to physicians. Many American TQM efforts have tended primarily to address the business and organizational aspects of hospitals and not
physicians and medical teams. Federal and state medical associations have
been slower to explore the potential of total quality management. In
contrast, the Joint Commission on Accreditation of Healthcare Organizations (a U.S. body) has been a leader in making quality a requirement for
accreditation as a hospital. In Canada, the Canadian Medical Association
(CMA) has included continuous quality improvement in its current philosophy and publications, and is offering physicians training in the tools
and techniques. And so, we in Canada have much to share with our
American colleagues concerning the inroads made with physician involvement and support for total quality management.

Given the U.S.'s high interest in the Canadian model of health care, it
may be that those hospitals in Canada that have become pioneers in total
quality management will illustrate for our neighbour to the south how
quality initiatives that focus on patient satisfaction, effective outcomes,
medical excellence, and cost effectiveness can work extremely well within
a universally accessible system. The September 1992 issue of *Consumer
Reports* summarizes for its American readers the five key principles of the
Canadian health care system under the Canada Health Act:

1. **Universality**. Everyone in the nation is covered.
2. **Portability**. People can move from province to province and from job to job (or onto the unemployment rolls) and still retain their health coverage.
3. **Accessibility**. Everyone has access to the system's health-care providers.
4. **Comprehensiveness**. Provincial plans cover all medically necessary treatment.
5. **Public administration**. The system is publicly run and publicly accountable.[15]

While Canada has traditionally felt the influence of U.S. business practices and economic strategies, it is *our* health-care system and Germany's that will likely be major influences on President Clinton and U.S. policy makers as they seek ways to improve access to health care for all Americans. If Canada can succeed in delivering accessible and high-quality health care across such a vast and disparate country, currently using about nine per cent of GNP, surely the U.S.'s 14 per cent can be put to more effective use.

Indeed, as Canadian hospitals experience positive achievements with total quality management and add these benefits to our more cost-effective system overall, we may find that we have in certain health care institutions a valuable export commodity — treatment and care to U.S. patients at less cost than, but equal in quality to, what they can get at home.

Strategies of total quality management may be the key to enabling the United States and Canada to share the search for health care system solutions that work. This is not to suggest that the U.S. will likely create a system identical to Canada's or to any other country's. What is paramount for the U.S. is the a more equitable health care system, one that will improve the level of health and health care of its citizens. Because of the economic and social links of the two countries, a healthier U.S. cannot help but benefit Canada economically in the long run.

WHAT WILL THE TQM HOSPITAL OF THE FUTURE LOOK LIKE?
We must not overlook the predictable chance of failure of organizations attempting total quality management. As mentioned in Chapter One, some indicators in the business industry are that seven out of ten have failed. A recent article in the *Globe and Mail* "Report on Business"

(January 2, 1993), organizational consultant David Bratton of London, Ontario, says people are drawn to fads. "I have my Andy Warhol theory of management concepts," he says. "What is hot now will be colder than a wet dog in six months. People say, 'I think I should TQM my company because everyone else is.'"

In that same article, Brian Harrison, president of A.T. Kearney Canada, says, "We see a lot of companies where TQM is in place but not understood. People pick one aspect like employee empowerment. They announce a cultural change, then train everybody and frequently produce nothing." There are many potential pitfalls in the development of a strategy of implementing TQM, and more stories are beginning to appear as to why it is unachievable. A simple analysis is that they don't understand the magnitude of the change required by leaders and by individuals in organizations, and, ultimately, the total transfiguration of the organization.

There have been many strategies suggested by health care professionals, health care policy-makers, and communities of measures to help create a health care system that will meet the needs of the future and maintain the high quality expected by all citizens. Many of these ideas, such as greater emphasis on health promotion and disease prevention, hospital outreach, and so forth have a lot of merit. But change in health care does not happen through good ideas alone. Current resource constraints are going to dictate that any change of direction for health care be supported by facts and figures on the viability of such change both in the short term and in the long term.

The tools and methods of total quality management can help provide those facts and figures. They offer reliable ways of gathering and analysing data, as well as being solidly based on the "designed in" concept of listening to customers and meeting their needs. In other words, total quality management may well make the difference between hospital programs or community initiatives that can be validated by data and results, and those that either fail or remain in the realm of ideas or conjecture.

It is unrealistic to think that within this decade, or even into the next century, we are going to see any significant increases in health care funding. Even if it did become possible to obtain huge resource increases in hospitals, it is unlikely that these increases would result in better levels of health for the population. For developed countries, our overall longevity and health status is about as good as it gets. As the ethicist Daniel Callahan has noted in his book *What Kind of Life?*, immortality is not an achievable health care goal.

This is not to ignore that there are some glaring gaps in health care delivery or in the health status of groups within populations — among the poor or among aboriginal peoples, for example. However, it is not increased resources that will create new solutions, but the rethinking and reallocation of already existing resources. Total quality management can help hospitals and communities do that.

Hospitals in future will be smaller, with fewer inpatient beds than is now the case. Downsizing is the order of the day and has already begun to happen, although we have not been able to come up with adequate strategies to cope with it. The emphasis on ambulatory care will increase greatly, particularly as new developments in technology enable more procedures and treatments to be conducted on an outpatient basis. As I mentioned in Chapter Two, we are at the end of the era of hospitalization, and we have not yet come to terms with the implications of this change for the direction of health care. Canadians have not accepted that *not* being in a hospital bed is best for some treatments. What is needed is greater public awareness of the possibility that good quality care can occur outside the hospital.

If the downsized hospitals and related health organizations of the future adopt a total quality management culture, then these smaller organizations will be more focused, more efficient, and more in tune with the needs of the communities they serve. A hospital in the process of taking on total quality management, such as St. Joseph's, is, granted, only a beginning step in refashioning the health care system. But if procedures and processes within our hospitals are effectively co-ordinated across the organization rather than departmentally, and if hospital care is carried out with a minimum of wasted resources and achieves both high quality and high patient/staff satisfaction, the stage will have been set for a further evolution into the community.

The customer focus which is at the heart of total quality management will help create ways for both hospitals and communities to assure themselves that health care resources are being used well. The TQM hospital of the future will play a key role in identifying and implementing health care processes that are effective not just within the hospital but within the community. A greater outpatient emphasis as a beginning will require that hospitals and communities create more effective linkages with each other and become close partners in delivering care to communities.

Hospitals and communities must work together to develop a realistic systems approach that will serve us in future. For example, health policy in Canada currently directs a great deal of attention toward the development of effective strategies for long-term care to accommodate the large numbers of baby boomers who, as they age, will have increased needs for care. We must be vigilant that we do not create an enormous and complex infrastructure that does not have the flexibility to downsize itself to adequately reflect the needs of the future *smaller* generation of elderly.

Accountability is another issue that must be addressed in a health system committed to total quality. If hospitals are going to work closely with communities to create health care that is responsive to communities' needs, and if communities are going to have input into how health needs will be met, I foresee that eventually hospitals and communities will relate to each other under a governance model based within regions rather than through the type of centralized governance that now exists from health ministries.

Hospitals of the future must transcend their traditional emphasis on treating illness and move toward a broader emphasis on promoting health and well-being; they must seek to heal, as well as cure or treat. Again, the rigorous focus on the customer as applied to health care will help keep this ideal of total well-being in the forefront of treatment and care. This same customer focus will be the key to hospitals and communities together being able to develop health care initiatives that are responsive to the specific setting in which they find themselves — whether we are talking about a large academic teaching hospital in an urban centre such as St. Joseph's, a community hospital serving a combination urban/rural area, or a small health facility in an isolated northern community.

Enabled people and empowered teams will characterize the successful organization. In *Zapp! The Lightning of Empowerment,* Byham and Cox paint a powerful picture of the typical manager as a white knight who charges in to slay the "dragons" of daily work life. This white knight, though well-intentioned, fails to realize that staff want to and can solve problems. Byham and Cox write, "Without pausing to ask where the dragon might be, the knight dropped his visor, lowered the point of his lance, and charged into the smoke. Unfortunately, his visibility limited by the tiny slits in the visor, the knight galloped right past the dragon and speared two of the workers."[16]

At St. Joseph's we have widely distributed copies of *Zapp!* to stimulate managers to see an alternative model of themselves. One of the most striking changes is the view that managers guide or coach staff to see a bigger picture of where the organization is headed, so that decisions are made and problems solved by staff. The learning organization of the future is deeply committed to the development of people and the unleashing of their inner power.

Max DePree, in *Leadership Is an Art,* describes a CEO not as the captain of the ship nor as the social convenor but rather as the designer. This concept is extended into Senge's thinking as he describes the architectural nature of the leader's role, that is to design the organization. Clearly CEOs must go beyond day-to-day management, beyond the practice of being involved in much of the operations of an organization, beyond being the white knight. The CEO enables others to achieve goals within the context of the vision and values established by the organization.

The cross-functional CQI teams and program strategies will require that health care professionals of the future be able to see how their roles fit into a cross-functional context. Legislation that sets the standards of practice for many health professions and defines their professional and legal identities, has a tendency to compartmentalize the health care system, thus erecting a barrier against TQM; health professionals must not allow this to happen. Total quality management in health care also challenges all health professionals, as well as nonclinical staff, to perceive not only the service and care links each has with the other, but also to understand and appreciate the social elements of health — that is, seeing patients and their families in the context of the larger reality of economics, community support networks, and personal and community relationships.

The success of TQM will also depend to a great degree on how well physicians are integrated into the new paradigm of flatter organizations, better use of resources, and more hospital-community interaction. In particular, we are going to have to take a close look at how physicians are reimbursed under the current system and determine if it is the best way for the future. Total quality management as it applies to health care is not, as I have stressed, primarily aimed at cost containment. However, cost management is almost always a positive side effect of total quality management, particularly in the ability of TQM techniques to identify inefficiencies, redundancies, and waste.

Built into a fee-for-service model is the incentive to provide more and more services. Even though the majority of physicians decide upon medical interventions out of a desire to genuinely help and serve their patients, the fee-for-service model drives the impetus to do more and more work and can cause the ordering of increased numbers of diagnostic tests and treatments. No amount of supporting data from continuous quality improvement projects that make the case for what are and are not appropriate medical interventions will be totally successful in altering medical practice while a financial incentive to do more is in place.

In academic health centres particularly, where there is a compelling demand for specialists to do more to maintain the critical mass of patients, to justify the existence of particular treatment programs, or to help fund medical research, the fee-for-service model may well be playing a role in obstructing many effective quality solutions to the issue of rising costs in health care. It now makes more sense in these centres for physicians to be salaried rather than on fee-for-service. How physicians are paid will continue to be a thorny issue throughout most of this decade. We will need the best win-win quality strategies in place to help us deal with it.

Community health centres (CHCs) in Canada or Health-maintenance Organizations (HMOs) in the U.S. give us clues to solving the dilemma facing us. In all modesty, I perceive that I work no less hard as a salaried person — and the same is true for most of the staff — than do fee-for-service physicians. While the issue of incentives must not be lost, they must not be the only determinant in aligning the system.

The creation of a seamless health care system from the community to the hospital and back to the community, as well as the ability to come up with positive strategies addressing the complex questions of health professionals' legitimate standards and the reimbursement of the system's key players — the physicians — is a daunting vision indeed. But we must not let the enormity of the larger vision stop us from beginning to make key changes right now. Every time we do something to make our services to patients better, every time we come up with a process improvement that removes bureaucratic obstacles and enables health care professionals to do their jobs efficiently and compassionately, we are moving gradually toward achieving this larger vision of continued excellence, improved processes, and continued accessibility for health care. This systemic thinking by all health agencies holds the answers to our future.

If our hospitals and health care agencies do take on the challenges of total quality management, the result will be a considerable shift of our health care system in a positive new direction. But I hasten to suggest that this transformation, as sweeping as it is, will only be one phase in coming to terms with a much larger health care reality.

As they gather, use, and share data from a wide variety of continuous quality improvement strategies, the hospitals of the future will become better at what they do and better at using available health care resources. This will then lead us to the next big challenge: how to make fundamental choices about exactly what we will do. Increasingly, health care decision-making falls into the realm of ethics, not just economics. If we manage to achieve a health system where needless waste is recaptured and where treatment programs are designed for maximum effectiveness and efficiency, we will still have to deal with this issue of just what we are doing.

Tough Choices   Total quality management will help us manage the resources we already have and those we only *may* acquire in future (nothing is guaranteed). As I have mentioned, the days of unlimited availability of resources are long gone. Choices will have to be made about where we want our health resources to go. If, for example, as a society we decide that we want health care to be directed primarily to helping create a better future for the nation's children, then what resources do we direct to the care of the elderly? Will resources be used to benefit the greatest number of people, and if so, what becomes of medicine's propensity to attempt extraordinary measures to save individual lives? When does good care, expected care, become heroic medicine, which may not in the long run reap any benefits either to individuals or to society? What is health?

Ethical Dilemmas   The story of three-year-old Kristina D'Andrea, reported widely in Ontario newspapers throughout much of 1992, was a poignant example of the type of torturous ethical dilemmas that families, hospitals, and funding bodies increasingly will face in the health care system of the future. The London, Ontario tot, victim of a rare genetic disease that leads to death usually by the time the child reaches puberty, was to have a bone-marrow transplant at Toronto's Hospital for Sick Children. But because the procedure is considered highly experimental for children with Kristina's condition, the Hospital for Sick Children eventually decided not to perform the procedure because of its extremely limited capacity to accommodate bone-marrow transplants. The number of children for whom the prognosis was better and who were on the waiting list for the procedure had to take precedence, the hospital was reported to say.

The child's family then turned to several U.S. facilities that were experienced with the experimental procedure. Again, they were turned down by key practitioners of the procedure on the basis that physicians were not satisfied the child met certain criteria. Since one of the possible side effects of the procedure is damage to a child's mental abilities, medical professionals felt that in Kristina's case the problems created by treatment would be greater than the benefits. The Ontario Ministry of Health, through OHIP, initially also refused to fund the procedure to be done out of country.

The physicians' refusal and the Ministry of Health's stance prompted an angry public outcry from much of the London community and elsewhere, and OHIP reversed its decision. Eventually, physicians in Iowa agreed to perform the procedure, which unfortunately was unsuccessful in arresting the child's condition.

No one could hear about this family's plight and not be moved. Of those of us who are parents, who would not want to try everything possible to save a child? Yet the procedure in question was highly experimental and deemed not likely to succeed with this particular child. And, in fact, it did not. Should the procedure have been attempted using health care system funding resources? Moral dilemmas such as this will in future become far more frequent as new treatment approaches and new technology enter medical practice at a dizzying rate. To make such decisions as humanely as possible yet serve the health care system as a whole, we will need to do much more work in the area of treatment outcomes, appropriatenes of procedures, and resource allocation.

The achievement of total quality management in our hospitals will not spare us these difficulties of choice or the moral task of deciding upon the fundamental values we wish to affirm in health care and in Canadian society as a whole. We cannot have it all. But by an unyielding focus on the customer, by helping us discover the best processes by which to deliver care, by uncovering the root causes of health care service problems, and by identifying opportunities for continuous improvement, total quality management will lead us to discover ways to serve Canadians' health care needs in far more ways than we ever dreamed possible. It is the medicine needed for our health care system to begin to heal itself from within, and to enable our societies to create a better tomorrow for all.

Appendix

Work Process Analysis

Statistical tools are used to help staff understand processes as they are currently set up and to identify and measure the variation in processes so that improvement can be made. Commonly called the "Magnificent Seven" because of their wide application, these tools help transform complicated data into powerfully simple visual charts.

SEVEN TOOLS AND METHODS OF CONTINUOUS QUALITY IMPROVEMENT

Flow Chart

Cause and Effect Chart

Run Chart

Measures

Time ➡

Pareto Chart

*

Type

Control Chart

Measures

10%

0%

-10%

Measurement Time

Histogram

*

Measurement

Scatter Diagram

Variable 2

Variable 1

DR. W. EDWARDS DEMING

220

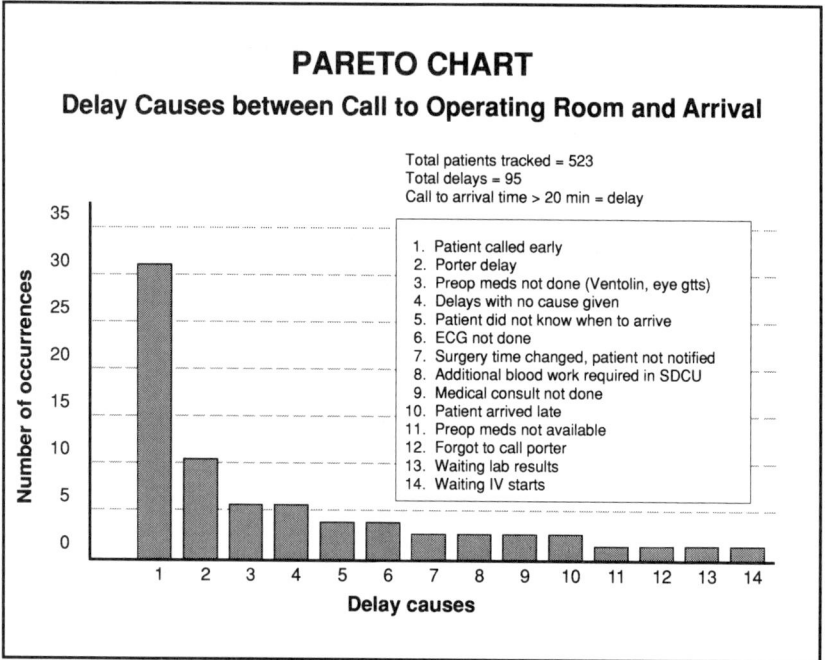

PARETO CHART
Delay Causes between Call to Operating Room and Arrival

Total patients tracked = 523
Total delays = 95
Call to arrival time > 20 min = delay

1. Patient called early
2. Porter delay
3. Preop meds not done (Ventolin, eye gtts)
4. Delays with no cause given
5. Patient did not know when to arrive
6. ECG not done
7. Surgery time changed, patient not notified
8. Additional blood work required in SDCU
9. Medical consult not done
10. Patient arrived late
11. Preop meds not available
12. Forgot to call porter
13. Waiting lab results
14. Waiting IV starts

Number of occurrences

Delay causes

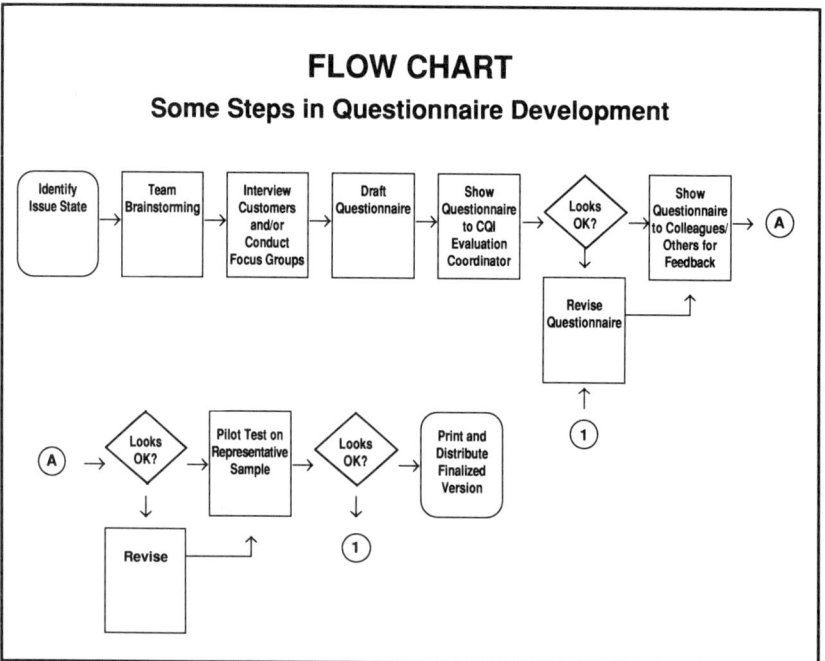

FLOW CHART
Some Steps in Questionnaire Development

Identify Issue State → Team Brainstorming → Interview Customers and/or Conduct Focus Groups → Draft Questionnaire → Show Questionnaire to CQI Evaluation Coordinator → Looks OK? → Show Questionnaire to Colleagues/ Others for Feedback → (A)

Revise Questionnaire

(1)

(A) → Looks OK? → Pilot Test on Representative Sample → Looks OK? → Print and Distribute Finalized Version

Revise

(1)

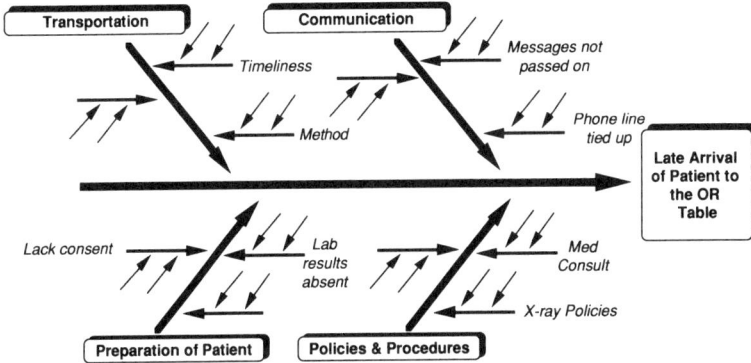

CAUSE AND EFFECT
Surgical Patient Flow

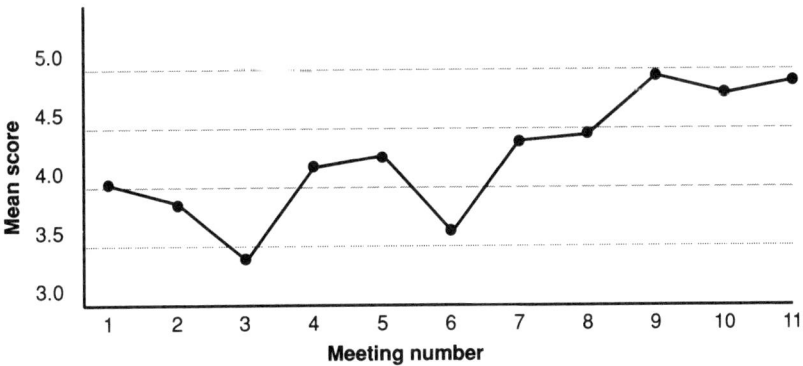

CONTROL CHART
Central Processing/OR Meeting Progress

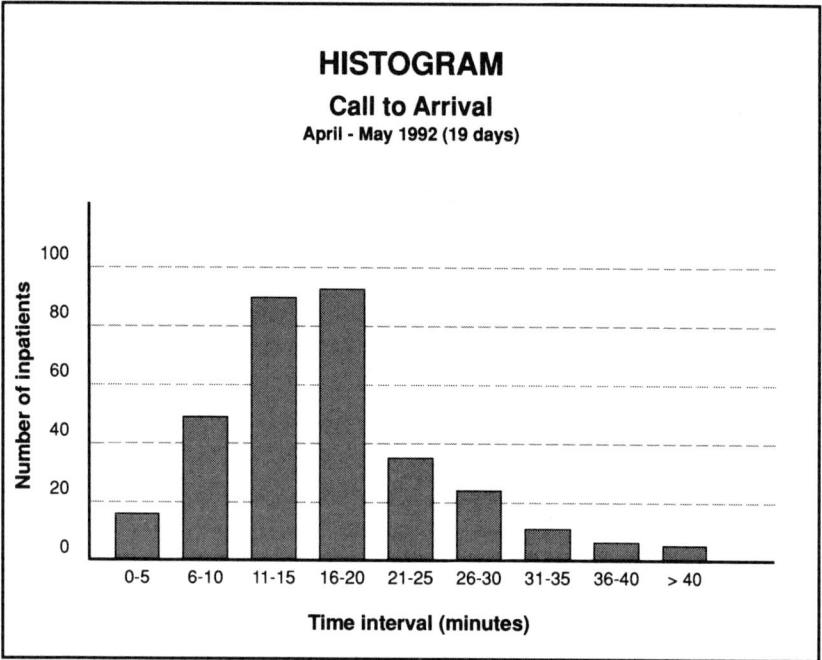

HISTOGRAM
Call to Arrival
April - May 1992 (19 days)

Endnotes

1 / A PRESCRIPTION FOR CHANGE

1. As reported in *The Globe and Mail*, April 25, 1992: "Total Quality Management Half Baked."
2. Quoted in *The Globe and Mail*, October 2, 1992: "Simply Put, Japanese Methods Aren't for All."
3. Donald Berwick; A. Blanton Godfrey; Jane Roessner, *Curing Health Care: New Strategies for Quality Improvement* (San Francisco & Oxford: Jossey-Bass Publishers, 1991), p. 158.
4. See Berwick, Chapter 7: "Implementing Successful Remedies," in *Curing Health Care*.
5. Total Health Expenditures as a percentage of GDP, Canada and the U.K. Source: Statistics Canada.
6. For example, see John Evans, "Illusions of Necessity: Evading Responsibility for Choice in Health Care," *Journal of Health Politics, Policy and Law* 10: 3 (Fall 1985).
7. Donald Berwick, *Curing Health Care*, p. 31.

2 / BEGINNING THE QUALITY JOURNEY

1. For example, see John Evans, "The Long Goodbye," *HSR: Health Sciences Research* 24: 4 (Oct. 1989).
2. Joel Barker in conversation with Joe Flower in "Don't Wait for the Crisis," *Healthcare Forum Journal*, November-December 1991.
3. Ibid.
4. Ibid.
5. International Quality Study, Health Care Industry Report, a joint project of Ernst & Young and American Quality Foundation, 1992, p. 47.
6. Ibid., p. 36
7. Ibid., pp. 1-2.
8. H. Eliasoph and P. Hassen, "VIP Streamlines Care and Reduces Length of Stay" in *Dimensions*, October 1986; and H. Eliasoph and P. Hassen, "Hospital Eyes Cataract Surgery," in *Health Management Forum*, Fall 1987.
9. Perry Danaan, "Position," *Warriors of the Heart* (Cooperstown, NY: Sunstone Publications, 1991).

3 / THE PHYSICIAN'S ROLE IN TOTAL QUALITY

1. Brent C. James, "How Do You Involve Physicians in TQM?" *Journal for Quality and Participation*, January-February 1991, p. 44.
2. Peter Cordy, "Continuous Quality Improvement: The Role of the Medical Staff," *Canadian Journal of Quality in Health Care*, March 1992, p. 6.

3. Donald Berwick, *Curing Health Care* (San Francisco/Oxford: Jossey-Bass Publishers, 1991), p. 151.
4. Ibid., p. 152.
5. Brent James, op. cit., p. 46-47.
6. Ibid., p. 44.
7. Donald Berwick, op. cit., p. 152.
8. Report of Dr. Martin Merry to St. Joseph's Health Centre Director of Total Quality Management, June 1992.
9. The Hospital Medical Records Institute (HMRI) has been analysing small area variations for Canada as well as other comparative Canadian data. See *Comparative Analysis of the HMRI Database*, compiled by Chris Helyar, HMRI, September 1992.
10. Klim McPherson, "Why Do Variations Occur?" in *The Challenges of Medical Practice Variations*, T. F. Andersen and G. Mooney, eds. (London: Macmillan, 1990).
11. MaryLou Harrigan, *Quality of Care: Issues and Challenges in the 90s: A Literature Review* (Stittsville, Ont.: Canadian Medical Association, 1992), p. 4.

4 / THE HOSPITAL AS A LEARNING ORGANIZATION

1. Quoted by Peter Senge in "The Leaders' New Work: Building Learning Organizations," *Sloan Management Review*, Fall 1990, p. 8. (Original article by B. Domain in *Fortune*, 3 July 1989, pp. 48-62.)
2. To explore this subject in more depth, read Robert Fritz, *The Path of Least Resistance* (New York: Ballantine, 1989), and *Creating* (New York: Ballantine, 1990).
3. A. Diane Moeller and Kathryn Johnson, "Shifting the Paradigm for Health Care Leadership," *Frontiers of Health Services Management*, 8: 3, pp. 28-29.
4. Peter F. Drucker, "The New Society of Organizations," *Harvard Business Review*, September-October 1992, pp. 95-96.
5. Ibid., p. 97.
6. Ibid., p. 101.

7 / THE NEW HEALTH CARE LEADER

1. From Joel Barker's video, *The Power of Vision*.
2. "The Cost of Quality," *Newsweek*, September 7, 1992.
3. Berwick, "TQM backlash prompts questions," *Hospitals*, June 5, 1992.
4. Warren Bennis, *On Becoming a Leader* (Menlo Park, CA: Addison-Wesley, 1989), p. 55.
5. Ibid., pp. 53, 71.
6. *The Globe and Mail*, October 13, 1992.

9 / WHAT DOES THE FUTURE HOLD?

1. International Quality Study, Health Care Industry Report, Ernst & Young and American Quality Foundation, 1992, p. 4.
2. Ibid., p. 5.
3. Ibid., pp. 53-54.
4. Ibid., p. 54.
5. Ibid., p. 56.
6. Leslie Greenwald, "Meaning in Numbers," *Health Management Quarterly*, Third Quarter 1992, p. 6.
7. "Wasted Health Care Dollars," *Consumer Reports*, July 1992, p. 436.
8. Leslie Greenwald, op. cit., p. 6.

9. *Consumer Reports,* July 1992, op. cit., p. 435.

10. Ibid., p. 435.

11. Ibid., p. 448.

12. U. Reinhardt, "Whither Private Health Insurance? Self-Destruction or Rebirth?" *Frontiers of Health Services Management* 9: 1, p. 7.

13. Donald Berwick, *Curing Health Care* (San Francisco & Oxford: Jossey-Bass, 1991), p. xv.

14. "Does Canada have the Answer?" *Consumer Reports,* September 1992, p. 580.

15. *Consumer Reports,* September 1992, p. 579.

16. William C. Byham, with Jeff Cox, *Zapp! The Lightning of Empowerment* (New York: Fawcett Columbine, 1988), p. 79.

Bibliography

BOOKS AND ARTICLES:

Albrecht, K., and Zemke, R. 1985. *Service America!* New York: Warner Books.

Anderson, C. A., and Daigh, R. D. 1991. "Quality mind-set overcomes barriers to success." *Healthcare Financial Management* 45(2): 20-22-22, 24, 26-32.

Barker, J. A. 1992. *Future Edge, Discovering the New Paradigms of Success.* New York: William Morrow.

Barth, D. 1989. "A four-step plan: Reaching total quality commitment." *Computer Healthcare* 10(6): 45-46, 49.

Bennis, W. 1989. *On Becoming a Leader.* Menlo Park, CA: Addison Wesley.

Berger, S., and Sudman, S. K. 1991. "Making total quality management work." *Healthcare Executive* (March/April): 22-25.

Berwick, D. M. 1989. "Continuous improvement as an ideal in health care." *New England Journal of Medicine* (January) 5: 53-56.

———. 1990. "Peer review and quality management: Are they compatible?" *Quality Review Bulletin* 16(7): 246-251.

Berwick, D. M., Godfrey, A.B. and Roessner, J. 1990. *Curing Health Care: New Strategies for Quality Improvement.* San Francisco: Jossey-Bass.

Block, P. 1987. *The Empowered Manager.* San Francisco: Jossey-Bass.

Burda, D. 1989. "AMI bonuses rise or fall based on quality." *Modern Healthcare* (April 7): 38.

———. 1989. "Prospects of quality measurement project excite the participating systems, alliances." *Modern Healthcare* (July 15): 40, 42, 44, 45.

———. 1988. "Providers look to industry for quality models." *Modern Healthcare* (July 15): 24-32.

———. 1989. "Quality college admits first hospital class." *Modern Healthcare* (January 20): 42.

————. 1991. "Total quality management becomes big business." *Modern Healthcare* (January 28): 25-29.

————. 1989. "Vt. hopes improved quality can control costs." *Modern Healthcare* (June 16): 38.

————. 1991. "The two (quality) faces of HCHP (Harvard Community Health Plan)." *Modern Healthcare* 21(ii): 28-29, 31.

Byham, W. C., and Cox, J. 1988. *Zapp! The Lightning of Empowerment*. New York: Fawcett Columbine.

Casalou, R. F. 1991. "Total quality management in health care." *Hospital Health Services Administration* 36(1): 134-146.

Cassidy, B. S. 1991. "Total quality management: an implementation strategy for excellence in the medical record department." *Topics in Health Records Management* 11(3): 44-57.

Clemmer, J. 1990. *Firing on All Cylinders*. Toronto: Macmillan.

Covey, S. R. 1991. *Principle-Centered Leadership*. New York: Summit.

Crosby, P. B. 1980. *The Eternally Successful Organization. The Art of Corporate Wellness*. Toronto: Penguin.

Crosby, P. B. 1979. *Quality Is Free: The Art of Making Quality Certain*. New York: McGraw-Hill.

Crosby, P. B. 1979. *Quality without Tears: The Art of Hassle-Free Management*. New York: McGraw-Hill.

Crosby, P. B. 1986. *Running Things: The Art of Making Things Happen*. New York: McGraw-Hill.

Crosby, P. B. 1989. *Let's Talk Quality: 96 Questions You Always Wanted to Ask Phil Crosby*. New York: McGraw-Hill.

Daigh, R. 1991. "How to start your own TQM (total quality management) program: Part one." *AOHA Today* 35(3): 6.

De Pree, M. 1989. *Leadership Is an Art*. New York: Bantam Doubleday.

Dixon, G. 1990. *Total Quality Handbook: The Executive Guide to the New American Way of Doing Business*. Minneapolis: Lakewood.

Donabedian, A. 1986. "Criteria and standards for quality assessment and monitoring." *Quality Review Bulletin* 12(3): 99-108.

Dowch, O. R. 1987. "What is quality care?" *The New England Journal of Medicine* (June 18): 1578-1580.

Drassard, M. 1988. *The memory jogger plus*. GOAL/QPC.

Gandz, J. 1990. "The Employee Empowerment Era." *Business Quarterly* 55(2): 74-79.

Gaucher, E. 1988. "Intrapreneurship: Tapping employee creativity." *The Journal of Nursing Administration* 18(12): 20-22.

Gelb, A. 1985. "Lessons from the Japanese." *The American Journal of Gastroenterology* 80(9): 738-742.

Gershon, M. 1991. "Statistical process control for the pharmaceutical industry." *Journal of Parenteral Science and Technology* 45(1): 41-50.

Ginnodo, W. L. 1991. "Management Style 2000." *Tapping the Network Journal* 2(1): 12-14.

Goman, C. K. 1991. *Managing for Commitment.* Oakville, Ontario: Reid.

Graham, N. O. 1990. *Quality assurance in hospitals: strategies for assessment and implementation.* 2nd ed. Rockville, MD: Aspen.

Green, D. K. 1991. "Quality improvement versus quality assurance?" *Topics in Health Records Management* 11(3): 58-70.

Green, J. 1988. "Change management: Hospitals are learning to make the most of change." *Modern Healthcare* (November 25): 20-22, 24, 26.

Hamson, N. (Ed.). 1991. "Visions of excellence in healthcare." *The Journal for Quality and Participation* (January/February).

Harrigan, M. L. 1992. *Quality of Care: Issues and Challenges in the 90's: A Literature Review.* Stittsville, Ont.: Canadian Medical Association.

Harrington, H. J. 1992. *The Improvement Process: How America's Leading Companies Improve Quality.* New York: McGraw-Hill.

Hart, C. W. L., Heskett, J. L., and Sasser, W. E., Jr. 1990. "The profitable art of service recovery." *Harvard Business Review* (July/August): 148-156.

Hauser, J. R., and Clausing, D. 1988. "The house of quality." *Harvard Business Review* (May/June): 63-73.

Hume, S. K. 1990. "Total quality management." *Health Progress* 71(8): 16-19.

Iglehart, J. K. 1988. "Japan's medical care system." *New England Journal of Medicine* 319(17): 807-812.

Iglehart, J. K. 1988. "Japan's medical care system: Part two." *New England Journal of Medicine* 319(17): 1166-1172.

Jaffe, D. T. and Scott, C. D. 1988. *Take This Job and Love It.* New York: Simon & Schuster.

Jensen, J. 1989. "Consumers consider quality in deciding on a hospital, but measurements differ." *Modern Healthcare* (March 10): 88.

Juran, J. M., and Gryna, F. M. (Eds.). 1988. *Juran's quality control handbook*. (4th ed.) New York: McGraw Hill.

Kelly, D., and Conner, D. R. 1979. "The emotional cycle of change." *The 1979 Annual Handbook for Group Facilitation*. San Diego, CA: University Associates.

Kimmel, R. B. 1989. "Agreeing on a definition of quality care may be healthcare's biggest challenge." *Modern Healthcare* (March 24): 37.

Kinlaw, D. C. 1991. *Developing Superior Work Teams: Building Quality and the Competitive Edge*. San Diego, CA: University Associates.

Kirk, R. 1988. *Healthcare Quality and Productivity: Practical Management Tools*. Rockville, MD: Aspen.

Kleefield, S., Churchill, W. W., and Laffel, G. 1991. "Quality improvement in a hospital pharmacy department." *Quality Review Bulletin* 17(5): 138-143.

Koska, M. T. 1990. "Adopting Deming's quality improvement ideas: A case study." *Hospitals* (July 5): 58-64.

————. 1990. "Case study: Quality improvement in a diversified health center." *Hospitals* 64(23): 38-39.

————. 1989. "CEO: Physician input vital to quality improvement." *Hospitals* 63(14): 22.

————. 1989. "Quality awareness pervades hospitals in '89." *Hospitals* 63(24): 26.

Kralovec, O. J. 3d., Huttner, C. A., and Dixon, M. D. 1991. "The application of total quality management concepts in a service-line cardiovascular program." *Nursing Administration Quarterly* 15(2): 1-8.

Kume, H. 1985. *Statistical Methods for Quality Improvement*. Tokyo: Association for Overseas Technical Scholarship.

Labovitz, G. 1991. "Beyond the total quality management mystique." *Healthcare Executive* (March/April): 15-17.

Laffel, G., and Blumenthal, D. 1989. "The case for using industrial quality management science in health care organizations." *JAMA* 262(20): 2869-2873.

Leebov, W., and Ersoz, C. J. 1991. *The Care Manager's Guide to Continuous Quality Improvement*. Chicago: American Hospital Publishing.

Lister, J. 1989. "Proposals for reform of the British National Health Service." *The New England Journal of Medicine* 320(13): 877-880.

Malcom Baldridge National Quality Award 1991 Application Guidelines.

Marszalek-Gaucher, E., and Coffey, R. J. 1990. *Transforming Healthcare Organizations: Visions and Actions for the Future*. San Francisco: Jossey-Bass.

Masters, F., and Schmele, J. A. 1991. "Total quality management: An idea whose time has come." *Journal of Nursing Quality Assurance* 5(4): 7-16.

McLaughlin, C. P., and Kaluzny, A. D. 1990. "Total quality management in health: Making it work." *Health Care Management Review* 15(3): 7-14.

McLaughlin, D. 1990. *Take the High Ground.* Tampa: Mancorn.

Meisenheimer, C. 1991. "The consumer: Silent or intimate player in the quality revolution?" *Holistic Nursing Practice* 5(3): 39-50.

————. 1992. *Improving Quality: A Guide to Effective Programs.* Rockville, MD: Aspen.

Melum, M. M. 1990. "Total quality management: Steps to success." *Hospitals* 64(23): 42, 44.

Merry, M. D. 1991. "Illusion vs. reality, TQM beyond the yellow brick road." *Healthcare Executive* (March/April): 18-21.

————. 1990. "Total quality management for physicians: Translating the new paradigm." *Quality Review Bulletin* 16(3): 101-105.

Mizuno, S. 1979. *Management for Quality Improvement: The 7 New QC Tools.* Cambridge, MA.: Productivity Press.

Moeller, A. D., and Johnson, K. 1992. "Shifting the Paradigm for Health Care Leadership." *Frontiers of Health Services Management* 8(3): 28-30.

Morgan, J. P., and Shields, D. W. 1990. "Using total quality management to improve patient relations programs." *Journal of Quality Assurance* 12(4): 38-41.

Moss Kanter, R. 1983. *The Change Masters.* New York: Simon & Schuster.

Naisbitt, J. 1982. *Megatrends: Ten New Directions Transforming Our Lives.* New York: Warner.

Naisbitt, J., and Aburdene, P. 1985. *Re-inventing the Corporation.* New York: Warner.

Nordlund, S. 1991. "Implementing total quality management programs in health care organizations." *Hospital Materials Management Quarterly* 12(4): 22-26.

Perry, L. 1988. "A suggestion: Solicit employees' ideas on quality." *Modern Healthcare* 18(38): 39.

Peters, T. 1987. *Thriving on Chaos: Handbook for a Management Revolution.* New York: Alfred A. Knopf.

Peters, T. J., and Waterman, R. H. 1982. *In Search of Excellence.* Cambridge, MA: Harper & Row.

Plsek, P. E. 1989. *Quality Improvement Tools.* Wilton, CT: Juran Institute.

Price, C. 1989. "Innovators and entrepreneurs: 1989." *Hospitals* (May 20): 40-54.

Quick, T. L. 1992. *Successful Team Building*. New York: AMACOM, Division of American Management Association.

Reich, R. B. 1987. "Entrepreneurship reconsidered: The team as hero." *Harvard Business Review* 65(3): 77-83.

Robinson, M. L. 1988. "Sneak preview: JCAHO's quality indicators." *Hospitals* (July 5): 38-43.

Robson, G. D. 1991. *Continuous process improvement: simplifying work flow systems*. Toronto: Maxwell Macmillan.

Roster, S. L. 1990. "Total quality improvement." *Journal of Quality Assurance* 12(4): 18-21.

Ruark-Hearst, M. 1991. "Cornerstones of health care in the nineties: Key constituencies debate propositions for collaborating in the quality revolution." *Quality Review Bulletin* 17(2): 60-65.

Ryan, K. D. and Oestreich, D. K. 1991. *Driving Fear Out of the Workplace*. San Francisco: Jossey-Bass.

Schaffer, R. H. and Thomson, H. A. 1992. *Successful Change Programs Begin with Results*. Harvard Business Review 70(1): 80-89.

Scholtes, P. R. 1988. *The Team Handbook*. Madison, WI: Jointer Associates.

Scott, C. D., and Jaffe, D. T. *Empowerment: A Practical Guide for Success*. Oakville, Ontario: Reid.

Spencer, L. J. 1989. *Winning through Participation: Meeting the Challenge of Corporate Change with the Technology of Participation*. Dubuque, IA: Kendall/Hunt.

Senge, P. M. 1990. *The Fifth Discipline*. New York: Doubleday.

Sherman, V. C. 1990. "Total management, not total quality management." *Journal of Quality Assurance* 12(4): 26-29.

Sinioris, M. E. 1990. "TQM (total quality management): The new frontier for quality and productivity improvement in health care." *Journal of Quality Assurance* 12(4): 14-17.

Talerico, M. 1991. "TQM (total quality management) is not a quick fix." *AOHA Today* 35(4): 6.

Thompson, R. E. 1991. "The six faces of quality: What total quality management really is." *Healthcare Executive* 6(2): 26-27.

Tichy, N. M., and Devana, M. A. 1990. *The Transformational Leaders*. Toronto: John Wiley and Sons.

Total Quality Newsletter Lakewood Publications, October 1991.

Vladeck, B. C. 1988. "Hospital prospective payment and the quality of care." *New England Journal of Medicine* 319(21): 1411-1413.

Walton, M. 1990. *The Deming Management Method.* New York: Putnam.

Wellins, R. S. 1991. *Empowered Teams: Creating Self-directed Work Groups that Improve Quality, Productivity and Participation.* San Francisco, CA: Jossey-Bass.

Wiggenhorn, W. 1990. "Motorola U: When training becomes an education." *Harvard Business Review* 68(4): 71-83.

Zenger, J. J., Musselwhite, E., Hurson, K. and Perrin, C. "Leadership in a Team Environment: The New American Manager." An Essay from Zenger-Miller, Inc.

VIDEOS

Barker, Joel Arthur. 1992. *Future Edge.* New York: William Morrow.

Barker, Joel Arthur. "The Business of Paradigms" and "The Power of Vision," *Discovering the Future Series.* New York: Chart House International Learning Corporation.

Berwick, Donald M., and Plsek. 1992. *Managing Medical Qualities: Quality Visions.*

Index